Dysbiosis

Jaime Ruiz-Tovar
Editor

Dysbiosis

Correlation between Changes in Microbiota and Pathology

Springer

Editor
Jaime Ruiz-Tovar
Health Sciences. San Juan de Dios School
of Nursing and Physical Therapy
Comillas Pontifical University
Paseo de la Habana 70B, Madrid, Spain

ISBN 978-3-031-65649-1 ISBN 978-3-031-65650-7 (eBook)
https://doi.org/10.1007/978-3-031-65650-7

This Springer imprint is published by the registered company Springer Nature Switzerland AG
The registered company address is: Gewerbestrasse 11, 6330 Cham, Switzerland

Contents

Microbiota. Microbiome. Applied Technologies and Omics Techniques Applied to the Microbiota. Metagenomics

1

Megan Trayling-Jiménez

1.1 What is the Microbiota and the Microbiome?

Microbiota refers to the community of microorganisms, primarily bacteria, but also there can be found viruses, fungi, archaea, and parasites that can be commensals, mutualists, or pathogens. The most common ones are *Staphylococcus aureus*, *Escherichia coli*, and *Candida albicans*, among others. These microorganisms play a crucial role in maintaining human health, as they participate in vital functions such as food digestion, vitamin B and K synthesis, immune system regulation, and protection against pathogens that are invading the body.

The human microbiota is found in different locations in the body, the most common ones being the gastrointestinal tract (intestines), skin, mouth, and upper respiratory and urogenital tracts. In the gastrointestinal tract, it is especially abundant in the large and small intestines. On the skin, it is found in the epidermis and hair follicles. In the mouth, bacteria can be found in the gums, teeth, and saliva. Lastly, in the upper respiratory tract, it is found in the nose and throat (Fig. 1.1).

On the other hand, the human microbiome is the complete set of genes and genetic material of all microorganisms in the body. This includes both beneficial and potentially harmful microorganisms. Beneficial microorganisms can be *Bifidobacteria* that contribute to fibre digestions and produce essential fatty acids or *Lactobacillus* that strengthen the immune system and improve digestion. On the other hand, harmful microorganisms can be *E. coli* that can cause gastrointestinal toxins and *Salmonella* that causes intestinal damage. The study of the human microbiome has revealed its influence on a wide range of medical conditions, from gastrointestinal diseases to neurological disorders and allergies. The balance between the microbiota and the microbiome is essential for optimal health. A dysbalance between the composition and function of the microbiota is called dysbiosis. It causes changes in the abundance of and diversity of the microorganisms that

M. Trayling-Jiménez (✉)
Department of Biomedicine, Universidad Alfonso X El Sabio, Madrid, Spain

J. Ruiz-Tovar (ed.), *Dysbiosis*, https://doi.org/10.1007/978-3-031-65650-7_1

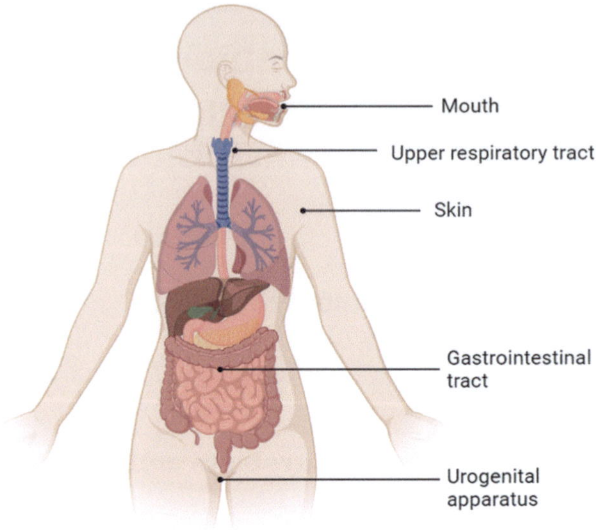

Fig. 1.1 Most common locations of human microbiota in the body

normally live in the intestine for example. This disequilibrium can be caused by different factors:

- Excessive use of antibiotics that can reduce microbial diversity and lead to the proliferation of resistant strains.
- Poor diet that promotes the growth of undesirable microorganisms and decrease the abundance of beneficial bacteria.
- Chronic stress can influence intestinal motility and barrier function.
- Excessive alcohol consumption which can damage the intestinal mucosa and allow pathogens to enter.
- Other diseases or gastrointestinal infections, lack of hygiene, and exposure to environmental contaminants like pesticides.
- Some drugs like non-steroidal anti-inflammatory drugs (NSAIDs) can cause gastrointestinal damage and affect the microbiota.

Restoring a proper balance in the microbiota is very important to treat problems associated with dysbiosis; this can be done with dietary modifications, the use of probiotics, and having healthy habits.

The microbiota has gained importance in recent scientific research because of its impact on human health. Furthermore, a close relationship has been found between the composition of the microbiota and a variety of medical conditions, such as obesity, autoimmune diseases, diabetes, and neurological disorders. This understanding has led to research aimed at microbiota therapies, including faecal transplantation, as well as a growing awareness of the importance of maintaining a microbiotic balance to promote optimal health.

Faecal transplantations involve the transfer of faecal material from a healthy donor to the intestine of a recipient with the aim of restoring or improving the intestinal microbiota. It seeks to restore a healthy balance in the recipient's microbiota by introducing beneficial microorganisms that compete and suppress the proliferation of harmful microorganisms, providing and effective alternative in cases of infections that are resistant to conventional treatments like antibiotics.

1.2 Technologies Applied to the Microbiota

Technologies applied to the microbiota have revolutionized the understanding of the microbial ecosystem in the human body. These advanced tools have enabled the analysis and characterization of the diversity, abundance, and functionality of microorganisms that make up the microbiota. Characterization of microbiota can be done through different types of approaches; the most common ones are:

1. Determining the composition of microorganisms through massive sequencing of the 16S rRNA gene using metataxonomics or metagenomics.
2. Identifying actively dividing bacteria through massive sequencing of cDNA from the 16S rRNA molecule, by active fraction metataxonomics.
3. Analyse their functional activity through identification and quantification of their metabolites using metabolomics.

Metataxonomics is a high-throughput process used to characterize the entire microbiota and create a metataxonomic tree that specifically focuses on taxonomic studies, revealing the relationship between the microbiome, and it also helps to characterize the composition and abundance of microbial communities. The process begins with the collection of biological samples, normally they are sourced from faeces, but also, they can be collected from saliva, skin, or other environments that host microbial communities from the microbiota. After the sample collection, the genetic material is extracted by sample disruption or cell lysis.

Subsequently, the highly informative 16S rRNA gene undergoes amplification via polymerase chain reaction (PCR) using universal primers, allowing for the identification of diverse microbial taxa due to its combination of conserved and variable regions.

The amplified DNA fragments then undergo high-throughput sequencing technologies like next-generation sequencing (NGS), generating extensive sequence data that encapsulates the microbial diversity present. Bioinformatic tools are used for comprehensive data analysis, including quality control, sequence filtering, and clustering for defining operational taxonomic units or exact sequence variants. Taxonomic assignment involves comparing obtained sequences to reference databases such as SILVA or the Ribosomal Database Project. The interpretation of the results provides information about the microbial community's structure, dynamics, responses to diverse conditions, and correlation with health or disease.

Active fraction metataxonomics provides functional information about the bacteria's direct or indirect impact on human health. To specifically identify active bacteria, the process involves extracting RNA from the sample, converting it to cDNA through retrotranscription, and subsequent sequencing, focusing only on dividing bacteria.

The main difference with metataxonomics is the starting genetic material. In active fraction metataxonomic is the 16S rRNA molecule. This targeted approach provides real-time insights into bacterial activity, emphasizing the dynamic role of active populations in influencing health.

Microfluidics offers a compact platform for in vitro simulation, cultivation, and manipulation of microbiota. This technology enables selective targeting and cultivation of key microbiota components and integrates culture, DNA extraction, amplification, and sequencing all in a single platform. This facilitates real-time monitoring of microbiota perturbations, allowing to do precise interventions. It also helps in researching guided antibiotic prescriptions for more targeted and effective treatments.

A microfluidic cell culture device is organs-on-a-chip; they mimic key aspects of the human's multicellular structures, interfaces, and microenvironments. In the context of intestinal studies, it allows a deep understanding of nutrient uptake, digestion, barrier function, drug metabolism, and infection mechanisms. The inclusion of analytical biosensors enables real-time assessment of physiological parameters. Organs-on-a-chip with hypoxia gradients support relevant microbial diversity, offering a valuable tool for studying microbiome-related therapeutics and infectious diseases (Fig. 1.2).

These chips consist of microscopic channels and cellular compartments that mimic physiological conditions of a specific organ. Cultivated human cells in these

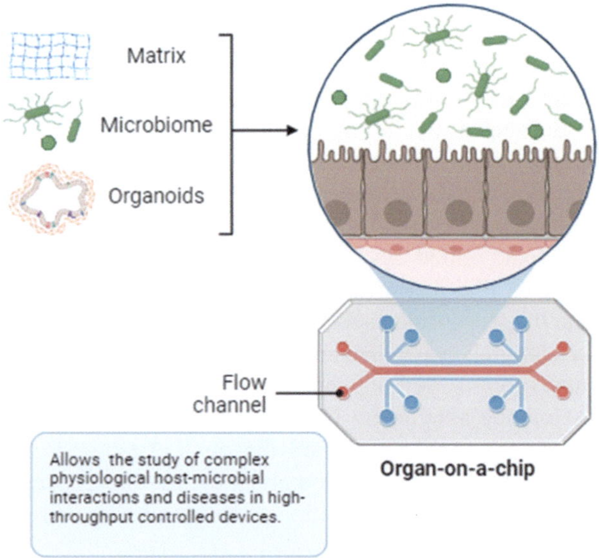

Fig. 1.2 Example of an organ-on-a-chip with its components

chips can experiment cellular interactions and responses to chemicals like what occurs in vivo. This technology involves the integration of cells, tissues, and micro-environmental factors in a system that allows the precise study of functions and responses at cellular level. They offer a valuable tool to investigate diseases, test drugs, and give a better understanding of human tissue responses and offer an efficient and ethical alternative to animal testing and accelerating drug development.

1.3 Omic Technologies Applied to the Microbiota

Omics include different technologies like genomics, transcriptomics, proteomics, and metabolomics; they play a crucial role in microbiotic research, providing different approaches to understand the composition and function of microbial communities.

- Genomics allows the identification of genes in the microbiota, showing diversity and potential functions.
- Transcriptomics analyses gene expression, indicating which genes are active at a given time.
- Proteomics focuses on the proteins produced, providing information about cellular activities.
- Metabolomics evaluates metabolites, offering a comprehensive view of metabolic interactions.

Together they allow a comprehensive understanding of the microbiota. Studying its taxonomic compositions and metabolic functions is essential for human health research and microbiota associated diseases.

Metabolomics is a discipline that focuses on the comprehensive study of the metabolites in organisms or biological system at a given time. In the microbiota, it is used to investigate the metabolic products produced by the interaction between the host and the microbial community in the gastrointestinal tract offering detailed information about metabolic activity and ongoing metabolic processes. Different techniques can be used:

- Nuclear magnetic resonance (NMR) is a non-destructive technique that gives information about structure and quantity of metabolites like organic acids and amino acids.
- Mass spectrometry (MS) is important for identifying and quantifying metabolites, using ionization methods like electrospray.
- MALDI-TOF is quick, and it efficiently profiles large biomolecules, accelerating the identification of metabolites.
- Secondary ion mass spectrometry (SIMS) offers subcellular resolution, allowing the analysis of metabolites within specific regions of microbial cells.

Its application in the microbiota allows to understand how microorganisms interact with the intestinal environment and how they affect the host's health. By identifying and quantifying specific metabolites, changes in the composition and function of the microbiota can be revealed, as well as their impact on health or associated diseases. It contributes to a more complete understanding of the mechanisms underlying host-microbiota relationships and offers valuable information for the development of therapeutic interventions based on microbiota modulation.

Metaproteomics is a high-throughput discipline that allows the comprehensive study of proteins present in a sample, whether of microbial or host origin. In the context of the microbiota, metaproteomics is used to obtain detailed information on the biological functions and activities of microbial communities in the intestine. This approach not only identifies the proteins present but also analyses their interactions, abundance levels, and post-translational modifications, providing a more complete view of microbial dynamics. Techniques used in metaproteomics include mass spectrometry (MS), nuclear magnetic resonance (NMR), microarrays, and protein analysis at the single cell level, allowing high-throughput characterization of proteins in the microbiota.

It is used to study the responses of the microbiota to changes in diet, the identification of potential biomarkers associated with gastrointestinal diseases, and the evaluation of the efficacy of therapeutic interventions aimed at modulating the composition and function of the microbiota. By providing a detailed view of proteins in the microbiota, it contributes significantly to the understanding of intestinal health and the development of personalized approaches for maintaining a proper microbiota balance.

Metatranscriptomics. This technique involves capturing, sequencing, and analysing the total mRNA or microRNA from a microbial ecosystem, providing insights into the active genes in the community. The process requires converting extracted RNA into complementary DNA (cDNA) through reverse transcriptase and primers, enabling the construction of libraries for subsequent sequencing.

In human gut microbiota, metatranscriptomics assumes a critical role by offering real-time glimpses into microbial activities and establishing correlations with the host's well-being. This technology serves as a powerful way to understand the complex correlation between the gut microbiota and the mucosal immune system (Fig. 1.3).

1.4 Metagenomics and Microbiota

Metagenomics is a field in genomics that focuses on the study of the collective genetic material of microbial communities in environmental samples, without the need to cultivate microorganisms individually.

In microbiota, metagenomics plays an essential role in providing a comprehensive approach to analyse the genetic and functional diversity of microbial communities. The method starts with DNA extraction, followed by library preparation and massive sequencing, using platforms like Illumina or Oxford Nanopore. The genetic

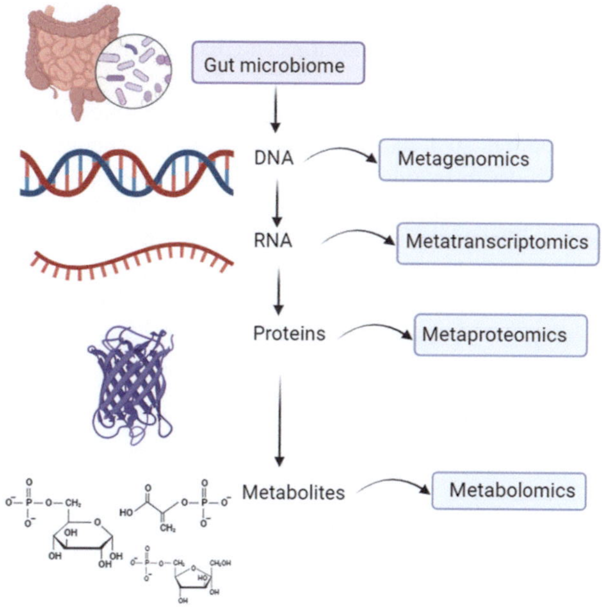

Fig. 1.3 Omic technologies applied to the gut microbiome with their extraction molecules

information obtained allows to explore the microbial composition, and it reveals potential functions, contributing to understanding of the influence of the microbiota in key processes like digestion, metabolism, and immune response.

It is similar to metataxonomics, but metagenomics provides a more complete view of genetic functions and diversity, while metataxonomy offers detailed information on the taxonomic composition of the microbiota. Metagenomics stands out for its ability to identify microorganisms that are present but also their genes and functions, giving valuable information for researchers.

Metagenomics has made some important discoveries, unravelling previously unknown microorganisms and giving information about their roles within the microbiome. Also, investigations about the microbiome with metagenomics have exposed its influence on digestion, metabolism, and immune function, with disruptions linked to a spectrum of diseases. It stands out for its capacity to capture the full genetic potential of the microbiome, offering insights into functional genes, metabolic pathways, and potential virulence factors.

The Human Microbiome Project (HMP) was an initiative led by the National Institutes of Health (NIH) that exemplifies the power of metagenomics. Launched in 2007, its main objective was to characterize the microbial diversity present in different sites of the human body and understand how the microbiota impacts health and disease. To carry out this microbiota research, HMP used metagenomics, using next-generation sequencing to analyse microbial DNA present in samples from various anatomical sites, such as the mouth, skin, intestines, and other areas. This pioneering project provided a comprehensive catalogue of microbial genes, identifying thousands of species and revealing the surprising genetic diversity of the human microbiota. Additionally, the project identified microbial patterns associated with various health conditions and diseases, from gastrointestinal disorders to metabolic diseases.

In addition, metagenomics offers distinct advantages over other 'omics' approaches such as metatranscriptomics or metaproteomics. While metatranscriptomics focuses on RNA expression and metaproteomics on protein analysis, metagenomics provides a comprehensive knowledge of the genomic potential of the entire microbial community. This inclusive approach allows for the identification of functional genes, metabolic pathways, and potential virulence factors. Functional metagenomics is a type of metagenomics that involves the direct cloning and expression of DNA fragments from microbiota samples that leads to the discovery of novel enzymes and metabolic pathways.

1.5 Conclusion

The microbiota and the microbiome are complex communities of microorganisms that play essential roles in human health, influencing processes like digestion and immune regulation. Advanced technologies, such as metagenomics and other omics techniques, have revolutionized the understanding of these systems by enabling detailed analysis of their genetic diversity, transcriptomics, proteomics, and metabolomics.

This advance has highlighted the critical importance of maintaining a proper balance in the microbiota, as imbalances, known as dysbiosis, can contribute to various medical conditions. From the Human Microbiome Project to innovative therapies such as faecal transplantations, advanced research offers promising pathways towards personalized interventions and discoveries that redefine the relationship between the microbiota and human health.

Additionally, omics technologies have revealed the complexity of microbial interactions at the molecular level, identifying the microbiota as a key player in the modulation of the immune system, nutrient synthesis, and response to various diseases. This in-depth knowledge has not only driven advances in the diagnosis and treatment of associated diseases but also lays the foundation for personalized health approaches based on microbiota modulation. Continued research in this field promises to open new perspectives for understanding the complex relationship between microorganisms and human health, paving the way towards more precise therapies and preventive strategies.

Suggested Readings

1. Abubucker S, Segata N, Goll J, Schubert AM, Izard J, Cantarel BL, Rodriguez-Mueller B, Zucker J, Thiagarajan M, Henrissat B, White O, Kelley ST, Methé B, Schloss PD, Gevers D, Mitreva M, Huttenhower C. Metabolic reconstruction for metagenomic data and its application

to the human microbiome. PLoS Comput Biol. 2012;8(6):e1002358. https://doi.org/10.1371/journal.pcbi.1002358.

2. Ajayi A, Jolaiya T, Smith S. Evolving technologies in gastrointestinal microbiome era and their potential clinical applications. J Clin Med. 2020;9(8):2565. https://doi.org/10.3390/jcm9082565.
3. Barh D, Blum K, Madigan MA, editors. OMICS: biomedical perspectives and applications. Boca Raton: CRC Press; 2017.
4. Cassotta M, Forbes-Hernández TY, Calderón Iglesias R, Ruiz R, Elexpuru Zabaleta M, Giampieri F, Battino M. Links between nutrition, infectious diseases, and microbiota: emerging technologies and opportunities for human-focused research. Nutrients. 2020;12(6):1827. https://doi.org/10.3390/nu12061827.
5. Dalal N, Jalandra R, Sharma M, Prakash H, Makharia GK, Solanki PR, Singh R, Kumar A. Omics technologies for improved diagnosis and treatment of colorectal cancer: technical advancement and major perspectives. Biomed Pharmacother. 2020;131:110648. https://doi.org/10.1016/j.biopha.2020.110648.
6. Daliri EB-M, Ofosu FK, Chelliah R, Lee BH, Oh D-H. Challenges and perspective in integrated multi-omics in gut microbiota studies. Biomol Ther. 2021;11(2):300. https://doi.org/10.3390/biom11020300.
7. del Campo-Moreno R, Alarcón-Cavero T, D'Auria G, Delgado-Palacio S, Ferrer-Martínez M. Microbiota en la salud humana: técnicas de caracterización y transferencia. Enferm Infecciosas y Microbiol Clin. 2018;36(4):241–5. https://doi.org/10.1016/j.eimc.2017.02.007.
8. Eloe-Fadrosh EA, Rasko DA. The human microbiome: from symbiosis to pathogenesis. Annu Rev Med. 2013;64(1):145–63. https://doi.org/10.1146/annurev-med-010312-133513.
9. Gosalbes MJ, Durbán A, Pignatelli M, Abellan JJ, Jiménez-Hernández N, Pérez-Cobas AE, Latorre A, Moya A. Metatranscriptomic approach to analyze the functional human gut microbiota. PLoS One. 2011;6(3):e17447. https://doi.org/10.1371/journal.pone.0017447.
10. Hardouin P, Chiron R, Marchandin H, Armengaud J, Grenga L. Metaproteomics to decipher CF host-microbiota interactions: overview, challenges and future perspectives. Genes. 2021;12(6):892. https://doi.org/10.3390/genes12060892.
11. Heinner G. Hacia la medicina personalizada: implicancias de las ciencias básicas y las 'ómicas' en la práctica clínica. Rev Peru de Med Exp y Salud Publica. 2015;32(4):629–32. http://www.scielo.org.pe/scielo.php?script=sci_arttext&pid=S1726-46342015000400001
12. Human Microbiome Project. Nih.gov. n.d.; Retrieved 8 December 2023, from https://commonfund.nih.gov/hmp
13. Izard J. In: Izard J, Rivera M, editors. Metagenomics for microbiology. Amsterdam: Elsevier Science; 2014.
14. Jovel J, Patterson J, Wang W, Hotte N, O'Keefe S, Mitchel T, Perry T, Kao D, Mason AL, Madsen KL, Wong GK-S. Characterization of the gut microbiome using 16S or shotgun metagenomics. Front Microbiol. 2016;7:459. https://doi.org/10.3389/fmicb.2016.00459.
15. Kiousi DE, Rathosi M, Tsifintaris M, Chondrou P, Galanis A. Pro-biomics: omics technologies to unravel the role of probiotics in health and disease. Adv Nutr. 2021;12(5):1802–20. https://doi.org/10.1093/advances/nmab014.
16. Lagier J-C, Dubourg G, Million M, Cadoret F, Bilen M, Fenollar F, Levasseur A, Rolain J-M, Fournier P-E, Raoult D. Culturing the human microbiota and culturomics. Nat Rev Microbiol. 2018;16(9):540–50. https://doi.org/10.1038/s41579-018-0041-0.
17. Mannaa M, Han G, Seo Y-S, Park I. Evolution of food fermentation processes and the use of multi-omics in deciphering the roles of the microbiota. Foods. 2021;10(11):2861. https://doi.org/10.3390/foods10112861.
18. Marchesi JR, Ravel J. The vocabulary of microbiome research: a proposal. Microbiome. 2015;3(1):1–3. https://doi.org/10.1186/s40168-015-0094-5.
19. Martín R, Miquel S, Langella P, Bermúdez-Humarán LG. The role of metagenomics in understanding the human microbiome in health and disease. Virulence. 2014;5(3):413–23. https://doi.org/10.4161/viru.27864.

20. Mehrian-Shai R, Reichardt JKV. Genomics is changing personal healthcare and medicine: the dawn of iPH (individualized preventive healthcare). Hum Genomics. 2015;9(1):1–2. https://doi.org/10.1186/s40246-015-0052-0.
21. Mutreja A. Microbial genomics. In: Kumar D, Antonarakis S, editors. Medical and health genomics. Amsterdam: Elsevier; 2016. p. 101–6.
22. NIH Human Microbiome Project. Hmpdacc.org. n.d.; Retrieved 8 December 2023, from https://hmpdacc.org/
23. Petrosino JF. Human Microbiome Project. Baylor College of Medicine. n.d.; Retrieved 8 December 2023, from https://www.bcm.edu/departments/molecular-virology-and-microbiology/research/human-microbiome-project
24. Segal JP, Mullish BH, Quraishi MN, Acharjee A, Williams HRT, Iqbal T, Hart AL, Marchesi JR. The application of omics techniques to understand the role of the gut microbiota in inflammatory bowel disease. Ther Adv Gastroenterol. 2019;12:175628481882225. https://doi.org/10.1177/1756284818822250.
25. Smith MI, Turpin W, Tyler AD, Silverberg MS, Croitoru K. Microbiome analysis—from technical advances to biological relevance. F1000 Prime Rep. 2014;6:51. https://doi.org/10.12703/p6-51.
26. Tomasello G, Mazzola M, Jurjus A, Cappello F, Carini F, Damiani P, Gerges GA, Zeenny MN, Leone A. The fingerprint of the human gastrointestinal tract microbiota: a hypothesis of molecular mapping. J Biol Regul Homeost Agents. 2017;31(1):245–9. https://pubmed.ncbi.nlm.nih.gov/28337900/
27. Turnbaugh PJ, Ley RE, Hamady M, Fraser-Liggett CM, Knight R, Gordon JI. The human microbiome project. Nature. 2007;449(7164):804–10. https://doi.org/10.1038/nature06244.
28. Ullah I, Yang L, Yin F-T, Sun Y, Li X-H, Li J, Wang X-J. Multi-omics approaches in colorectal cancer screening and diagnosis, recent updates and future perspectives. Cancers. 2022;14(22):5545. https://doi.org/10.3390/cancers14225545.
29. van den Elsen LWJ, Poyntz HC, Weyrich LS, Young W, Forbes-Blom EE. Embracing the gut microbiota: the new frontier for inflammatory and infectious diseases. Clin Transl Immunol. 2017;6(1):e125. https://doi.org/10.1038/cti.2016.91.
30. Wang W-L, Xu S-Y, Ren Z-G, Tao L, Jiang J-W, Zheng S-S. Application of metagenomics in the human gut microbiome. World J Gastroenterol: WJG. 2015;21(3):803. https://doi.org/10.3748/wjg.v21.i3.803.
31. Yang J, Pu J, Lu S, Bai X, Wu Y, Jin D, Cheng Y, Zhang G, Zhu W, Luo X, Rosselló-Móra R, Xu J. Species-level analysis of human gut microbiota with metataxonomics. Front Microbiol. 2020;11:2029. https://doi.org/10.3389/fmicb.2020.02029.
32. Zhang X, Li L, Butcher J, Stintzi A, Figeys D. Advancing functional and translational microbiome research using meta-omics approaches. Microbiome. 2019;7(1):154. https://doi.org/10.1186/s40168-019-0767-6.

Prebiotics, Probiotics, Symbiotics and Postbiotics. Nutrition and Microbiota

2

Jaime Ruiz-Tovar and Carolina Llavero

2.1 Introduction

The gastrointestinal (GI) tract is primarily responsible for digestion, enabling the absorption of nutrients. However, the gut is involved in other relevant functions, such as the regulation of energy homeostasis or the immune response [1]. Energy balance is regulated by the central nervous system and peripheral receptors that detect the arrival of nutrients in the diet and the shortage of nutrients in cases of fasting. These peripheral receptors are located in the gut itself, the pancreas and adipose tissue [2]. From these peripheral tissues, energy status is communicated to brain centres via endocrine and nerve signals, which determine the appropriate response to adapt food intake, nutrient partitioning, and nutrient catabolism accordingly [2, 3].

The gastrointestinal tract represents a physical but selective barrier of defence against external pathogens, while maintaining neutrality towards micro-organisms belonging to the saprophytic flora. The intestinal mucosal barrier is composed of different layers: the lumen, the mucus layer, the intestinal epithelium and the lamina propria [1, 4]. The mucus layer harbours a large diversity of commensal micro-organisms, known as gut microbiota, and their respective metabolites. The mucus layer is composed mainly of water and mucins (glycosylated proteins secreted by goblet cells) and confers a semi-permeable environment, allowing selective passage of substances from the intestinal lumen to the epithelial cells, but preventing the entry of micro-organisms, both saprophytes and pathogens [1, 4, 5].

J. Ruiz-Tovar (✉)
San Juan de Dios Foundation, Madrid, Spain

Health Sciences, Department. San Juan de Dios School of Nursing and Physical Therapy, Comillas Pontifical University, Madrid, Spain
e-mail: jruiztovar@comillas.edu

C. Llavero
Department of Nursery, Henares University Hospital, Madrid, Spain

J. Ruiz-Tovar (ed.), *Dysbiosis*, https://doi.org/10.1007/978-3-031-65650-7_2

Different types of epithelial cells constitute the intestinal epithelium. The enterocytes are the cells responsible for maintaining structural integrity and regulating absorption; the goblet cells secrete mucus; Paneth cells produce the antimicrobial peptides; M cells are involved in immunity responses, and the enteroendocrine cells release hormones for endocrine and paracrine communication between the gut and diverse organs [1, 4, 6]. A rupture in the mucosal or epithelial barriers might allow pathogens and bacterial products to disseminate mainly through the portal vein circulation to peripheral organs [7]. Consequently, the gut barrier regulates metabolic homeostasis, whose function is compromised in metabolic diseases such as obesity, type 2 diabetes (T2DM), or malnutrition disorders [7–10].

2.2 Composition and Nutritional Functions of Microbiota

Trillions of microorganisms, most of them bacteria, inhabit the human gut in a symbiotic relationship with the host. Microbiota participates in the regulation of host defences, by training the immune system through antigen exposure. The absence of gut microbiota might result in insufficient mesenteric lymph nodes and incapacity to produce antibodies [11]. Furthermore, microbiota takes an active role in the digestion of nutrients, as dietary indigestible products are degraded by bacteria, converting them in absorbable substances or fibre to conform faeces [12]. During digestion, the gut microbiota produces short-chain fatty acids (SCFA) from the metabolism of dietary fibre, which are important not only to maintain the epithelial barrier but also to keep immune homeostasis [13]. SCFA are correlated with better glycaemic and lipid profiles and improved metabolism of macro- and micronutrients [14, 15].

An adequate balance between the main bacterial phyla (*Bacteroidetes, Firmicutes, Actinobacteria, Proteobacteria, Verrucomicrobia*) and the diversity of bacterial groups is essential to maintain the homeostasis in the entire organism and reduces the risk of appearance of diverse diseases affecting different organs and systems, not exclusively the gastrointestinal tract [15]. The dysbalance in the microbiota is called dysbiosis. Contributors to dysbiosis include antibiotics, drugs, alcohol, stress, genetic susceptibility and inadequate diets [15–17]. A short period of exposure to any of these factors is enough to induce marked alteration in the microbiota.

The gut microbiota has demonstrated to be an active part of fat storage regulation [18]. Thus, inadequate diets, mostly high-fat diets, are closely related to dysbiosis. Diet-induced obesity promotes dysbiosis mainly by increasing *Firmicutes/Bacteroidetes* [15, 17, 19–30]. As a consequence of this dysbiosis, there is an increased capacity to accumulate energy from food and the generation of an inflammatory environment [31]. In terms of the changing pattern of species present in the gut, there is a high prevalence of gram-negative bacteria, producing lipopolysaccharide (LPS), which will activate Toll-like receptors (TLRs). This will promote the activation of nuclear factor kappa β (NF-κB)-dependent transcription programmes for several proinflammatory cytokines, contributing to colonic inflammation and causing damage to the epithelial barrier [23, 24, 26, 29–36]. Inadequate diets also alter hepatic bile acid (BA) secretion, which are converted to secondary BA by the microbiota within the colon. Secondary BA play a role in fat digestion and control the gut microbiome (increasing *Firmicutes*/*Bacteroidetes* ratio) while reducing the risk of bowel inflammation [7]. However, at chronically high levels, secondary BA are associated with colonic inflammation and intestinal barrier dysfunction [7, 37, 38]. Long-term high-fat diets are able to increase LPS levels in circulation, inducing LPS-dependent systemic inflammation, the so-called metabolic endotoxemia, which might initiate/contribute to the metabolic sequelae of obesity [19].

Different disorders in *Akkermansia muciniphila* have been also associated with nutritional pathologies. A decrease in their populations has been correlated with obesity. Extracellular vesicles from *Akkermansia muciniphila* are able to reduce weight gain in high-fat diets, by improving tight-junctions and thus decreasing intestinal permeability [39]. Glucose-enriched diets were shown to induce loss in tight-junction proteins and increased gut barrier permeability assayed by plasma LPS levels [27]. Therefore, usual diets of developed countries (high sugar and HFD) are associated with a pattern of dysbiosis (increased *Firmicutes*/*Bacteroidetes* ratio) and an eventual increase in the intestinal inflammatory response and barrier disruption [40–43]. In women with obesity, the permeability of the small intestine is increased, as measured by the lactulose/mannitol excretion, and correlated positively with waist/abdominal perimeter and with the homeostatic model assessment of insulin resistance (HOMA-IR) [44]. Moreover, gut permeability was also positively associated with visceral adiposity in healthy overweight women. In contrast, high fibre intake is related to lower amounts of *Proteobacteria*, increased SCFA and weight loss in overweight and obese subjects [45–48], improving gut barrier integrity, as measured by lactulose/mannitol and polyethylene glycol excretion [49–51]. Altogether, these data show the powerful role of the diet itself in the fast modulation of gut microbiota and barrier permeability. Some dietary factors have been linked to a balanced microbiome and restored gut function, such as fibre and polyunsaturated fatty acids. Customized dietary interventions can be actually designed, as the contribution of specific foods on gut microbiota and modulation of inflammation is starting to be elucidated [52]. Omega-3 supplementation seems to restore the *Firmicutes*/*Bacteroidetes* ratio and increase SCFA production (by increasing *Prevotella* and *Bacteroides*), thus being associated with better metabolic outcomes [53, 54]. Cereals, vegetables and fish are closely associated with microbiota balance, reduced inflammation and increased SCFA production [55]. On the other hand, environmental factors such as air pollutants, heavy metals, pesticides and other contaminating foods can also alter the gut microbiota [56–60]. Beneficial gut microbiota modulators are probiotic supplementation, including *Lactobacillus* spp. and *Bifidobacterium* spp., reducing intestinal inflammation and barrier disruption [8, 61]. Exercise training is also a potent modulator of the gut microbiota, by decreasing the *Firmicutes*/*Bacteroidetes* ratio and improving intestinal inflammation in sedentary obese adults [62].

2.3 Consequences of Dysbiosis and Inflammation on Gut Function and Nutritional Status

As previously mentioned, the gut communicates with other organs either through nervous connections or endocrine signaling, to regulate energy balance [2]. The vagus nerve regulates the gut-brain-liver connection, controlling glucose homeostasis by suppressing hepatic glucose production upon nutrient sensing in the duodenum and jejunum [63, 64]. Furthermore, the GI tract secretes diverse hormones, while nutrient digestion and absorption stimulate the secretion of anorexigenic signals (GLP-1, CCK, and PYY); nutrient deficits stimulate ghrelin secretion to promote feeding [65]. The synchronicity between neuronal and humoral signals traveling across the crossroads of the gut-brain axis will govern overall energy homeostasis.

A healthy microbiota regulates gut signal secretion by the production of SCFA from dietary fibre digestion [14]. SCFA stimulate GLP-1 and PYY secretion, favouring an anorexigenic effect and stimulating incretin release. Altogether, these factors contribute to a beneficial metabolic effect [66, 67]. Secondary BA also stimulate GLP-1 secretion [68]. Other metabolites derived from bacterial metabolism, such as indole derived from bacteria-mediated tryptophan metabolism, are stimulants of gut hormone secretion. Indole also regulates GLP-1 secretion [69].

Furthermore, the gut microbiota produces several neurotransmitters (acetylcholine, dopamine, serotonin and γ-aminobutyric acid (GABA)) that can act in the enteric nervous system or in brain centres [70]. Additionally, SCFA induce a direct stimulatory effect on the vagus nerve, independently of enteric neurotransmitter release [71].

SCFA production is also altered by dysbiosis, as the latter induces the loss of butyrate-producing bacteria [72–74]. Consequently, the SCFA-mediated gut hormone secretion, such as GLP-1, may change. In obese subjects, the *Lactobacillus* spp. reduction has been associated with decreased GLP-1 response [75]. Furthermore, circadian alterations of microbiota participate in the regulation of GLP-1 production [76]. Loss in SCFA production might also impair the vagal response since butyrate contributes to vagal afferent stimulation [71]. Consequently, a reduction in vagal innervation to the brain is reduced [77].

Circulating GLP-1 and GLP-2 levels have been shown to be decreased under inflammatory conditions [78–80]. Interestingly, GLP-1 agonists have demonstrated to improve the clinical expression of inflammatory bowel disease, by reducing the release of inflammatory cytokines [81]. Clinical pilot studies using GLP-2 analogues have demonstrated higher remission rates in patients with Crohn's disease [82–84]. In contrast, ghrelin levels were reported to be increased in patients with Crohn's disease and ulcerative colitis [85]. On the other hand, subjects who underwent vagotomy have an increased risk of developing inflammatory bowel disease, highlighting the immunomodulatory effect of the vagus nerve activity [86, 87].

Prebiotic supplementation has shown to ameliorated gut inflammation and intestinal barrier integrity, while restoring GLP-1 and GLP-2 levels [88–90].

2.4 Prebiotics, Probiotics, Symbiotics and Postbiotics

Prebiotics are a class of functional foods, defined as non-digestible food ingredients that are utilised by the gut microbiota. They stimulate the growth of one or more strains of bacteria present in the intestinal tract and modify their composition and activity, thereby achieving an improvement in the health and well-being of the host. Prebiotics are capable of enriching the gut microbiota with strains of bacteria belonging to the genera *Lactobacillus and Bifidobacterium* [88, 89]. The gut microbiota generates fermented products from prebiotics, such as SCFA (acetate, propionic acid, butyric acid). Prebiotics are generally carbohydrates, but there is recent evidence that certain polyphenols may possess prebiotic characteristics. Among prebiotics, dietary fibre, fructo-oligosaccharides and inulin can be included [90].

Probiotics are added live organisms that remain active in the gut in sufficient quantity to alter the host gut microbiota, both by implantation and colonisation. They can have beneficial effects when ingested in sufficient quantities [91].

Symbiotics refer to foods containing a mixture of prebiotics and probiotics. As a general rule, they should contain a prebiotic component that supports the effect of the associated probiotic food, such as the association of oligofructans with *Bifidobacteria*. Symbiotic foods are generally dairy products in liquid form similar to a yoghurt [92].

Postbiotics are soluble factors (metabolic products), secreted by live bacteria, or released after bacterial lysis providing a beneficial effect. Postbiotic can be also called paraprobiotics, as these are immobilised probiotics, which when ingested can present biological responses and restore intestinal homeostasis in a similar way to probiotics [93]. Postbiotics are gaining attraction in the last years because of their indication to subjects with low tolerance to probiotics, mostly in children and in immunocompromised patients. They seem to have similar beneficial properties as live probiotics with fewer risk of adverse effects. Postbiotics release bacterial components, such as lipoteichoic acids, peptidoglycans, or exopolysaccharides, whose properties imply immunomodulating effects and inhibition against pathogens, performing their beneficial effect modulating the immune response [94].

There is increasing evidence of the use of all these compounds as therapeutic tools for different diseases, especially those where dysbiosis has been demonstrated. They have also been used in inflammatory diseases, since, as mentioned above, dysbiosis can induce a chronic pro-inflammatory state and the restoration of a balanced microbiota can reduce this inflammatory response, not only at the digestive level but also implying multiple organs and systems [92].

Postbiotics are newly emerging and there is little evidence about their efficacy. Some clinical studies have shown that postbiotics might play a role in general health and well-being and can improve host immune function similar to probiotics [95]. Postbiotics can induce changes in the altered gut microbial composition, which is associated with elevated levels of innate and acquired immunity biomarkers. Furthermore, postbiotics also seem to exhibit antioxidant effects [96]. Postbiotics have been evaluated in small study sizes and seem to be beneficial for clinical applications, like gastrointestinal diseases (bloating, diarrhoea, …), upper respiratory tract infections, asthma, inflammatory bowel diseases, type 2 diabetes, atopic dermatitis or influenza viruses infection [95, 96].

2.5 Conclusion

Many of the components of the diet (fibres, macro-, and micronutrients) are digested by the microbiota, and most of the physiological functions of the gut are regulated by the metabolites resulting from such modifications. Usual diets in developed countries with a lipid and sugar overload and potentially also contaminated with residual levels of chemicals and pollutants induce rapid and marked dysbiosis (alterations in gut microbiota composition and its metabolites) that may be accompanied by gut inflammation and barrier disruption. This dysbiosis leads to increased levels of pro-inflammatory factors in the gut.

The gut microbiota has a modulatory effect on vagal tone and the production of GLP-1, PYY, serotonin, through SCFA production, having a relevant impact in gut-brain communication. Dysbiosis hampers gut hormone production. However, there is still a long way to understand the relation between gut microbiota and impaired energy balance.

References

1. Farré R, Fiorani M, Abdu Rahiman S, Matteoli G. Intestinal permeability, inflammation and the role of nutrients. Nutrients. 2020;12:1185.
2. Badman MK, Flier JS. The gut and energy balance: visceral allies in the obesity wars. Science. 2005;307(5717):1909–14.
3. Yi C-X, Tschöp MH. Brain–gut–adipose-tissue communication pathways at a glance. Dis Model Mech. 2012;5(5):583–7.
4. Vancamelbeke M, Vermeire S. The intestinal barrier: a fundamental role in health and disease. Expert Rev Gastroenterol Hepatol. 2017;11:821–34.
5. Jakobsson HE, Rodríguez-Piñeiro AM, Schütte A, Ermund A, Boysen P, Bemark M, Sommer F, et al. The composition of the gut microbiota shapes the colon mucus barrier. EMBO Rep. 2015;16:164–77.
6. Chelakkot C, Ghim J, Ryu SH. Mechanisms regulating intestinal barrier integrity and its pathological implications. Exp Mol Med. 2018;50:1–9.
7. Portincasa P, Bonfrate L, Khalil M, Angelis MD, Calabrese FM, D'Amato M, et al. Intestinal barrier and permeability in health obesity NAFLD. Biomedicines. 2021;10:83.
8. Kang Y, Kang X, Yang H, Liu H, Yang X, Liu Q, et al. Lactobacillus acidophilus ameliorates obesity in mice through modulation of gut microbiota dysbiosis and intestinal permeability. Pharmacol Res. 2022;175:106020.
9. Rehman AU, Siddiqui NZ, Farooqui NA, Alam G, Gul A, Ahmad B, et al. Morchella esculenta mushroom polysaccharide attenuates diabetes and modulates intestinal permeability and gut microbiota in a type 2 diabetic mice model. Front Nutr. 2022;9:984695.
10. Xie F, Xu H-F, Zhang J, Liu X-N, Kou B-X, Cai M-Y, et al. Dysregulated hepatic lipid metabolism and gut microbiota associated with early-stage NAFLD in ASPP2-deficiency mice. Front Immunol. 2022;13:974872.
11. Round JL, Mazmanian SK. The gut microbiome shapes intestinal immune responses during health and disease. Nat Rev Immunol. 2009;9:313–23.

12. Ge Y, Ahmed S, Yao W, You L, Zheng J, Hileuskaya K. Regulation effects of indigestible dietary polysaccharides on intestinal microflora: an overview. J Food Biochem. 2021;45:e13564.
13. Di Tommaso N, Gasbarrini A, Ponziani FR. Intestinal barrier in human health and disease. Int J Environ Res Public Health. 2021;18:12836.
14. Müller M, Hernández MAG, Goossens GH, Reijnders D, Holst JJ, Jocken JWE, et al. Circulating but not faecal short-chain fatty acids are related to insulin sensitivity, lipolysis and GLP-1 concentrations in humans. Sci Rep. 2019;9:12515.
15. Weiss GA, Hennet T. Mechanisms and consequences of intestinal dysbiosis. Cell Mol Life Sci. 2017;74:2959–77.
16. Buttó LF, Haller D. Dysbiosis in intestinal inflammation: cause or consequence. Int J Med Microbiol. 2016;306:302–9.
17. Malesza IJ, Malesza M, Walkowiak J, Mussin N, Walkowiak D, Aringazina R, et al. High-fat, western-style diet, systemic infammation, and gut microbiota: a narrative review. Cells. 2021;10:3164.
18. Bäckhed F, Ding H, Wang T, Hooper LV, Koh GY, Nagy A, et al. The gut microbiota as an environmental factor that regulates fat storage. Proc Natl Acad Sci. 2004;101:15718–23.
19. Cani PD, Amar J, Iglesias MA, Poggi M, Knauf C, Bastelica D, et al. Metabolic endotoxemia initiates obesity and insulin resistance. Diabetes. 2007;56:1761–72.
20. Cani PD, Bibiloni R, Knauf C, Waget A, Neyrinck AM, Delzenne NM, Burcelin R. Changes in gut microbiota control metabolic endotoxemia-induced infammation in high-fat diet-induced obesity and diabetes in mice. Diabetes. 2008;57:1470–81.
21. Garidou L, Pomié C, Klopp P, Waget A, Charpentier J, Aloulou M, et al. The gut microbiota regulates intestinal CD4 T cells expressing RORγt and controls metabolic disease. Cell Metab. 2015;22:100–12.
22. Turnbaugh PJ, Bäckhed F, Fulton L, Gordon JI. Diet induced obesity is linked to marked but reversible alterations in the mouse distal gut microbiome. Cell Host Microbe. 2008;3:213–23.
23. Kim KA, Gu W, Lee IA, Joh EH, Kim DH. High fat diet-induced gut microbiota exacerbates infammation and obesity in mice via the TLR4 signaling pathway. PLoS One. 2012;7(10):e47713.
24. Lam YY, Ha CWY, Campbell CR, Mitchell AJ, Dinudom A, Oscarsson J, et al. Increased gut permeability and microbiota change associate with mesenteric fat infammation and metabolic dysfunction in diet-induced obese mice. PLoS One. 2012;7:e34233.
25. Heisel T, Montassier E, Johnson A, Al-Ghalith G, Lin YW, Wei LN, et al. High-fat diet changes fungal microbiomes and interkingdom relationships in the murine gut. mSphere. 2017;2:e00351–e417.
26. Velázquez KT, Enos RT, Bader JE, Sougiannis AT, Carson MS, Chatzistamou I, et al. Prolonged high-fat-diet feeding promotes nonalcoholic fatty liver disease and alters gut microbiota in mice. World J Hepatol. 2019;11:619–37.
27. Do MH, Lee E, Oh M-J, Kim Y, Park H-Y. High-glucose or -fructose diet cause changes of the gut microbiota and metabolic disorders in mice without body weight change. Nutrients. 2018;10:761.
28. Lin H, An Y, Hao F, Wang Y, Tang H. Correlations of fecal metabonomic and microbiomic changes induced by high-fat diet in the pre-obesity state. Sci Rep. 2016;6:21618.
29. De La Serre CB, Ellis CL, Lee J, Hartman AL, Rutledge JC, Raybould HE. Propensity to high-fat diet-induced obesity in rats is associated with changes in the gut microbiota and gut inflammation. Am J Phys. 2010;299:G440–8.
30. Sen T, Cawthon CR, Ihde BT, Hajnal A, DiLorenzo PM, de La Serre CB, Czaja K. Diet-driven microbiota dysbiosis is associated with vagal remodeling and obesity. Physiol Behav. 2017;173:305–17.
31. Turnbaugh PJ, Ley RE, Mahowald MA, Magrini V, Mardis ER, Gordon JI. An obesity-associated gut microbiome with increased capacity for energy harvest. Nature. 2006;444:1027–31.

32. Ding S, Chi MM, Scull BP, Rigby R, Schwerbrock NMJ, Magness S, et al. High-fat diet: bacteria interactions promote intestinal inflammation which precedes and correlates with obesity and insulin resistance in mouse. PLoS One. 2010;5:e12191.
33. Barbara G, Barbaro MR, Fuschi D, Palombo M, Falangone F, Cremon C, et al. Inflammatory and microbiota-related regulation of the intestinal epithelial barrier. Front Nutr. 2021;8:718356.
34. Johnson AMF, Costanzo A, Gareau MG, Armando AM, Quehenberger O, Jameson JM, Olefsky JM. High fat diet causes depletion of intestinal eosinophils associated with intestinal permeability. PLoS One. 2015;10:e0122195.
35. Kuipers EN, Kantae V, Maarse BCE, van den Berg SM, van Eenige R, Nahon KJ, et al. High fat diet increases circulating endocannabinoids accompanied by increased synthesis enzymes in adipose tissue. Front Physiol. 2018;9:1913.
36. Cuddihey H, MacNaughton WK, Sharkey KA. Role of the endocannabinoid system in the regulation of intestinal homeostasis. Cell Mol Gastroenterol Hepatol. 2022;14:947–63.
37. Li J-Y, Gillilland M, Lee AA, Wu X, Zhou S-Y, Owyang C. Secondary bile acids mediate high-fat diet-induced upregulation of R-spondin 3 and intestinal epithelial proliferation. JCI Insight. 2022;7:e148309.
38. Zeng H, Safratowich BD, Cheng WH, Larson KJ, Briske Anderson M. Deoxycholic acid modulates cell-junction gene expression and increases intestinal barrier dysfunction. Molecules. 2022;27:723.
39. Chelakkot C, Choi Y, Kim DK, Park HT, Ghim J, Kwon Y, et al. Akkermansia muciniphila-derived extracellular vesicles influence gut permeability through the regulation of tight junctions. Exp Mol Med. 2018;50:e450.
40. Fajstova A, Galanova N, Coufal S, Malkova J, Kostovcik M, Cermakova M, et al. Diet rich in simple sugars promotes pro-inflammatory response via gut microbiota alteration and TLR4 signaling. Cells. 2020;9:2701.
41. Thaiss CA, Levy M, Grosheva I, Zheng D, Sofer E, Blacher E, et al. Hyperglycemia drives intestinal barrier dysfunction and risk for enteric infection. Science. 2018;359:1376–83.
42. Harte AL, Varma MC, Tripathi G, McGee KC, Al-Daghri NM, Al-Attas O, et al. High fat intake leads to acute postprandial exposure to circulating endotoxin in type 2 diabetic subjects. Diabetes Care. 2012;35:375–82.
43. Ley RE, Turnbaugh PJ, Klein S, Gordon JI. Human gut microbes associated with obesity. Nature. 2006;444:1022–3.
44. Teixeira TFS, Souza NCS, Chiarello PG, Franceschini SCC, Bressan J, Ferreira CL, Maria CGD. Intestinal permeability parameters in obese patients are correlated with metabolic syndrome risk factors. Clin Nutr. 2012;31:735–40.
45. Gummesson A, Carlsson LMS, Storlien LH, Bäckhed F, Lundin P, Löfgren L, et al. Intestinal permeability is associated with visceral adiposity in healthy women. Obesity. 2011;19:2280–2.
46. Brignardello J, Morales P, Diaz E, Romero J, Brunser O, Gotteland M. Pilot study: alterations of intestinal microbiota in obese humans are not associated with colonic infammation or disturbances of barrier function. Aliment Pharmacol Ther. 2010;32:1307–14.
47. David LA, Maurice CF, Carmody RN, Gootenberg DB, Button JE, Wolfe BE, et al. Diet rapidly and reproducibly alters the human gut microbiome. Nature. 2014;505:559–63.
48. Medawar E, Haange S-B, Rolle-Kampczyk U, Engelmann B, Dietrich A, Thieleking R, et al. Gut microbiota link dietary fiber intake and short-chain fatty acid metabolism with eating behavior. Transl Psychiatry. 2021;11:500.
49. Ott B, Skurk T, Hastreiter L, Lagkouvardos I, Fischer S, Büttner J, et al. Effect of caloric restriction on gut permeability, inflammation markers, and fecal microbiota in obese women. Sci Rep. 2017;7:11955.
50. Li T, Hui H, Hu C, Ma H, Yang X, Tian J. Multiscale imaging of colitis in mice using confocal laser endomicroscopy, light-sheet fluorescence microscopy, and magnetic resonance imaging. J Biomed Opt. 2019;24:1–8.
51. Quero G, Saccomandi P, Kwak J-M, Dallemagne B, Costamagna G, Marescaux J. Modular laser-based endoluminal ablation of the gastrointestinal tract: in vivo dose-effect evaluation and predictive numerical model. Surg Endosc. 2019;33:3200–8.

52. Chen T, Long W, Zhang C, Liu S, Zhao L, Hamaker BR. Fiber-utilizing capacity varies in Prevotella-versus Bacteroides dominated gut microbiota. Sci Rep. 2017;7:2594.
53. Fu Y, Wang Y, Gao H, Li D, Jiang R, Ge L, Tong C, et al. Associations among dietary omega-3 polyunsaturated fatty acids, the gut microbiota, and intestinal immunity. Mediat Inflamm. 2021;2021:8879227.
54. Li X, Guo J, Ji K, Zhang P. Bamboo shoot fiber prevents obesity in mice by modulating the gut microbiota. Sci Rep. 2016;6:32953.
55. Bolte LA, Vich Vila A, Imhann F, Collij V, Gacesa R, Peters V, Wijmenga C, et al. Long-term dietary patterns are associated with pro-inflammatory and antiinflammatory features of the gut microbiome. Gut. 2021;70:1287–98.
56. Mousavi SE, Delgado-Saborit JM, Adivi A, Pauwels S, Godderis L. Air pollution and endocrine disruptors induce human microbiome imbalances: a systematic review of recent evidence and possible biological mechanisms. Sci Total Environ. 2022;816:151654.
57. Jiang P, Yuan G, Jiang B, Zhang J, Wang Y, Lv H, et al. Effects of microplastics (MPs) and tributyltin (TBT) alone and in combination on bile acids and gut microbiota crosstalk in mice. Ecotoxicol Environ Saf. 2021;220:112345.
58. Van den Brule S, Rappe M, Ambroise J, Bouzin C, Dessy C, Paquot A, Muccioli GG, Lison D. Diesel exhaust particles alter the profile and function of the gut microbiota upon subchronic oral administration in mice. Part Fibre Toxicol. 2021;18(1):7.
59. Alderete TL, Jones RB, Chen Z, Kim JS, Habre R, Lurmann F, et al. Exposure to traffic-related air pollution and the composition of the gut microbiota in overweight and obese adolescents. Environ Res. 2018;161:472–8.
60. Jerrett M, McConnell R, Wolch J, Chang R, Lam C, Dunton G, et al. Traffic related air pollution and obesity formation in children: a longitudinal, multilevel analysis. Environ Health. 2014;13(1):49.
61. Monteros MJM, Galdeano CM, Balcells MF, Weill R, De Paula JA, Perdigón G, Cazorla SI. Probiotic lactobacilli as a promising strategy to ameliorate disorders associated with intestinal infammation induced by a non-steroidal antiinflammatory drug. Sci Rep. 2021;11:571.
62. Motiani KK, Collado MC, Eskelinen J-J, Virtanen KA, Löyttyniemi E, Salminen S, et al. Exercise training modulates gut microbiota profile and improves endotoxemia. Med Sci Sports Exerc. 2020;52:94–104.
63. Chen J, Cheng M, Wang L, Zhang L, Xu D, Cao P, et al. A vagal-NTS neural pathway that stimulates feeding. Curr Biol. 2020;30:3986–3998.e5.
64. Wang PYT, Caspi L, Lam CKL, Chari M, Li X, Light PE, Gutierrez-Juarez R, Ang M, Schwartz GJ, Lam TKT. Upper intestinal lipids trigger a gut–brain–liver axis to regulate glucose production. Nature. 2008;452:1012–6.
65. Rosendo-Silva D, Matafome P. Gut–adipose tissue crosstalk: a bridge to novel therapeutic targets in metabolic syndrome? Obes Rev. 2021;22:e13130.
66. Larraufe P, Martin-Gallausiaux C, Lapaque N, Dore J, Gribble FM, Reimann F, Blottiere HM. SCFAs strongly stimulate PYY production in human enteroendocrine cells. Sci Rep. 2018;8:74.
67. Tolhurst G, Hefron H, Lam YS, Parker HE, Habib AM, Diakogiannaki E, et al. Short-chain fatty acids stimulate glucagon-like peptide-1 secretion via the G-protein-coupled receptor FFAR2. Diabetes. 2012;61:364–71.
68. Wei M, Huang F, Zhao L, Zhang Y, Yang W, Wang S, et al. A dysregulated bile acid-gut microbiota axis contributes to obesity susceptibility. EBioMedicine. 2020;55:102766.
69. Chimerel C, Emery E, Summers DK, Keyser U, Gribble FM, Reimann F. Bacterial metabolite indole modulates incretin secretion from intestinal enteroendocrine L cells. Cell Rep. 2014;9:1202.
70. Bonaz B, Bazin T, Pellissier S. The vagus nerve at the interface of the microbiota-gut-brain axis. Front Neurosci. 2018;12:49.
71. Lal S, Kirkup AJ, Brunsden AM, Thompson DG, Grundy D. Vagal afferent responses to fatty acids of different chain length in the rat. Am J Physiol Gastrointest Liver Physiol. 2001;281:G907–15.

72. Martin AM, Sun EW, Keating DJ. Mechanisms controlling hormone secretion in human gut and its relevance to metabolism. J Endocrinol. 2020;244:R1–R15.
73. Loper H, Leinen M, Bassof L, Sample J, Romero-Ortega M, Gustafson KJ, et al. Both high fat and high carbohydrate diets impair vagus nerve signaling of satiety. Sci Rep. 2021;11:10394.
74. DeGruttola AK, Low D, Mizoguchi A, Mizoguchi E. Current understanding of dysbiosis in disease in human and animal models. Inflamm Bowel Dis. 2016;22:1137–50.
75. Grasset E, Puel A, Charpentier J, Collet X, Christensen JE, Tercé F, Burcelin R. A specific gut microbiota dysbiosis of type 2 diabetic mice induces GLP-1 resistance through an enteric nondependent and gut-brain axis mechanism. Cell Metab. 2017;25:1075–1090.e5.
76. Martchenko SE, Martchenko A, Cox BJ, Naismith K, Waller A, Gurges P, et al. Circadian GLP-1 secretion in mice is dependent on the intestinal microbiome for maintenance of diurnal metabolic homeostasis. Diabetes. 2020;69:2589–602.
77. Kim JS, Kirkland RA, Lee SH, Cawthon CR, Rzepka KW, Minaya DM. Gut microbiota composition modulates inflammation and structure of the vagal afferent pathway. Physiol Behav. 2020;225:113082.
78. Cao H, Liu X, An Y, Zhou G, Liu Y, Xu M, et al. Dysbiosis contributes to chronic constipation development via regulation of serotonin transporter in the intestine. Sci Rep. 2017;7:10322.
79. Hunt JE, Holst JJ, Jeppesen PB, Kissow H. GLP-1 and intestinal diseases. Biomedicines. 2021;9:383.
80. Zatorski H, Sałaga M, Fichna J. Role of glucagon-like peptides in inflammatory bowel diseases—current knowledge and future perspectives. Naunyn Schmiedeberg's Arch Pharmacol. 2019;392:1321–30.
81. Moore BA, Pefer N, Pirone A, Bassiri A, Sague S, Palmer JM, et al. GLP-2 receptor agonism ameliorates infammation and gastrointestinal stasis in murine postoperative ileus. J Pharmacol Exp Ther. 2010;333:574–83.
82. Teduglutide Study Group, Buchman AL, Katz S, Fang JC, Bernstein CN, Abou-Assi SG. Teduglutide, a novel mucosally active analog of glucagon-like peptide-2 (GLP-2) for the treatment of moderate to severe Crohn's disease. Inflamm Bowel Dis. 2010;16:962–73.
83. Villumsen M, Schelde AB, Jimenez-Solem E, Jess T, Allin KH. GLP-1 based therapies and disease course of inflammatory bowel disease. eClinicalMedicine. 2021;37:100979. https://doi.org/10.1016/j.eclinm.2021.100979.
84. El-Salhy M, Hatlebakk JG, Hausken T. Possible role of peptide YY (PYY) in the pathophysiology of irritable bowel syndrome (IBS). Neuropeptides. 2020;79:101973.
85. El-Salhy M. Ghrelin in gastrointestinal diseases and disorders: a possible role in the pathophysiology and clinical implications. Int J Mol Med. 2009;24:727–32.
86. Mikami Y, Tsunoda J, Kiyohara H, Taniki N, Teratani T, Kanai T. Vagus nerve-mediated intestinal immune regulation: therapeutic implications of inflammatory bowel diseases. Int Immunol. 2022;34:97–106.
87. Liu B, Wanders A, Wirdefeldt K, Sjölander A, Sachs MC, Eberhardson M, Ye W, et al. Vagotomy and subsequent risk of inflammatory bowel disease: a nationwide register-based matched cohort study. Aliment Pharmacol Ther. 2020;51:1022–30.
88. Rojas-Renjifo K, Urrego-Restrepo LM, Ramírez-Navas JS. Prebiotics, their effect on patients with gastrointestinal diseases. Salutem Scientia Spiritus. 2022;8(3):99–111.
89. Teng PY, Kim WK. Review: roles of prebiotics in the intestinal ecosystem of broilers. Front Vet Sci. 2018;5:245.
90. Roberfroid M. Prebiotic effects: metabolic and health benefits. Br J Nutr. 2010;104(Suplemento S2):S1–S63.
91. Olveira Fuster G, González-Molero I. Probiotics and prebiotics in clinical practice. Nutr Hosp. 2007;22(Suppl 2):26–34.
92. Cosier DJ, Lambert K, Neale EP, Probst Y, Charlton K. The effect of oral synbiotics on the gut microbiota and inflammatory biomarkers in healthy adults: a systematic review and meta-analysis. Nutr Rev. 2024;82:nuae002.

93. Aguilar-Toalá JE, Garcia-Varela R, Garcia HS, Mata-Haro V, González-Córdova AF, Vallejo-Cordoba B, Hernández-Mendoza A. Postbiotics: An evolving term within the functional foods field. Trends Food Sci Technol. 2018;75:105–14.
94. Popovic N. The influence of heat-killed enterococcus faecium BGPAS1-3 on the tight junction protein expression and immune function in differentiated Caco-2 cells infected with listeria monocytogenes ATCC 19111. Front Microbiol. 2019;10:412.
95. Pique N, Berlanga M, Minana-Galbis D. Health benefits of heat-killed (Tyndallized) probiotics: an overview. Int J Mol Sci. 2019;10:20.
96. Berni CR. Specific signatures of the gut microbiota and increased levels of butyrate in children treated with fermented Cow's Milk containing heat-killed lactobacillus paracasei CBA L74. Appl Environ Microbiol. 2017;19:83.

Microbiota and Neurodegenerative and Brain Diseases

3

Malena Martinez-Orive

3.1 Pathophysiological Bases

The microbiota is the immense set of all types of microorganisms (bacteria, viruses, fungi, protozoa, etc.) that inhabit the human body, presenting marked differences between all parts of the body depending on the physical-chemical characteristics of a given area. One of the most active branches of research today is the study of the gut-brain axis.

3.1.1 Gut-Brain Axis

The gut-brain axis is a nervous connection that communicates and allows the brain control motility and secretion in the digestive tract. Depending on its activity, it is classified within the autonomic nervous system (ANS), called the enteric nervous system (ENS). It is mainly identified by the vagus nerve, an innervation belonging to the parasympathetic ANS, and by neuronal networks located in the wall (Auerbach's plexus) and mucosa (Meissner's plexus) of the digestive tract. The Auerbach's plexus are nerve fibers arranged along and between the layers of muscle tissue in the walls of the digestive tract and control the motility of the digestive tract. The Meissner's plexus is located near the mucosa of the digestive tract, innervating endocrine and exocrine secretory glands, exerting control over digestive secretions. The gut-brain axis is a bidirectional neuronal communication pathway, which implies that the information circulating between the central nervous system (CNS) and the gastrointestinal tract (GI) each detect and transmit a response, establishing complementary functioning. The information sent by the CNS is in the form of neurotransmitters that circulate through the axons of the nerve fibers of the vagus nerve, which translates into a function of motility or hormonal secretion. The effects

M. Martinez-Orive (✉)
Department of Biomedicine, Universidad Alfonso X, Madrid, Spain

J. Ruiz-Tovar (ed.), *Dysbiosis*, https://doi.org/10.1007/978-3-031-65650-7_3

of the gut-brain axis are also influenced by some autonomic centers of the medulla oblongata and higher centers, such as the limbic system and nuclei of the hypothalamus. We must understand the CNS and the SNE as a team that requires communication and signals from both parties to guarantee survival. For example, when faced with threats, the fight-flight response is activated in the CNS, which emits a vasoconstriction signal in the arteries of the digestive system, controlled by the SNE, to reduce blood flow and divert it to vital organs and muscles. Another example in which they work hand in hand is in the control of appetite and satiety. The lateral hypothalamic nucleus (CNS) is known as the "appetite center" due to the existence of two different neuronal groups that balance the sensation of hunger and satiety. Orexigenic neurons promote the sensation of appetite by inhibiting anorexigenic neurons (satiety) through neuropeptide Y and activating the release of ghrelin (the hunger hormone) at the level of the stomach through the action of the SNE or gut-brain axis. In addition, responses occur such as increased release of gastric and intestinal secretion to visual and olfactory stimuli of food. The effect of dopamine on the limbic system causes a sensation of pleasure to be experienced when eating certain types of foods (Fig. 3.1).

A more necessary link for the gut-brain axis is the participation of the immune system. The immune system at the level of the large intestine is based mainly on mast cells, a type of polymorphonucleated cell sensitive to neurotransmitters from the CNS and the ENS itself. At the histological level of the wall of the large intestine, they are located in the lamina propria, a structure formed by proteins of the extracellular matrix, which delimits the intestinal mucosa from the luminal side of the intestine. Thanks to this strategic area, mast cells monitor sensory stimuli coming from the lumen and, if necessary, activate the immune response against antigens. Mast cells are a varied group of cells that can present different receptors on their cell membrane and participate in a wide range of actions, one of them being participation in the gut-brain axis by releasing chemicals such as histamine.

3.1.2 Neurotransmitters and Intestinal Microbiota

Due to advances in knowledge of the gut-brain axis in relation to the microbiota and in terms of functioning, it currently receives the more correct definition of microbiota-gut-brain axis. There are two main ways by which the microbiota modifies brain function: the vagus nerve and blood circulation. The microbiota uses the vagus nerve to send rapid signals to the brain; and on the other hand, it synthesizes molecules in its metabolism that act as precursors that travel through the blood circulation and modify the levels of these and other metabolites in the brain. Precursor molecules, such as tyrosine and tryptophan amino acids, together with the precursors L-DOPA and 5-HTP can be introduced into neurotransmitter synthesis cycles and give rise to dopamine, glutamate, GABA, or serotonin. These are common neurotransmitters that regulate the excitation or inhibition of neurons in the brain, but when they are synthesized in excess due to the extra contribution of precursors from an altered microbiota, they end up generating an imbalance in neurotransmitter

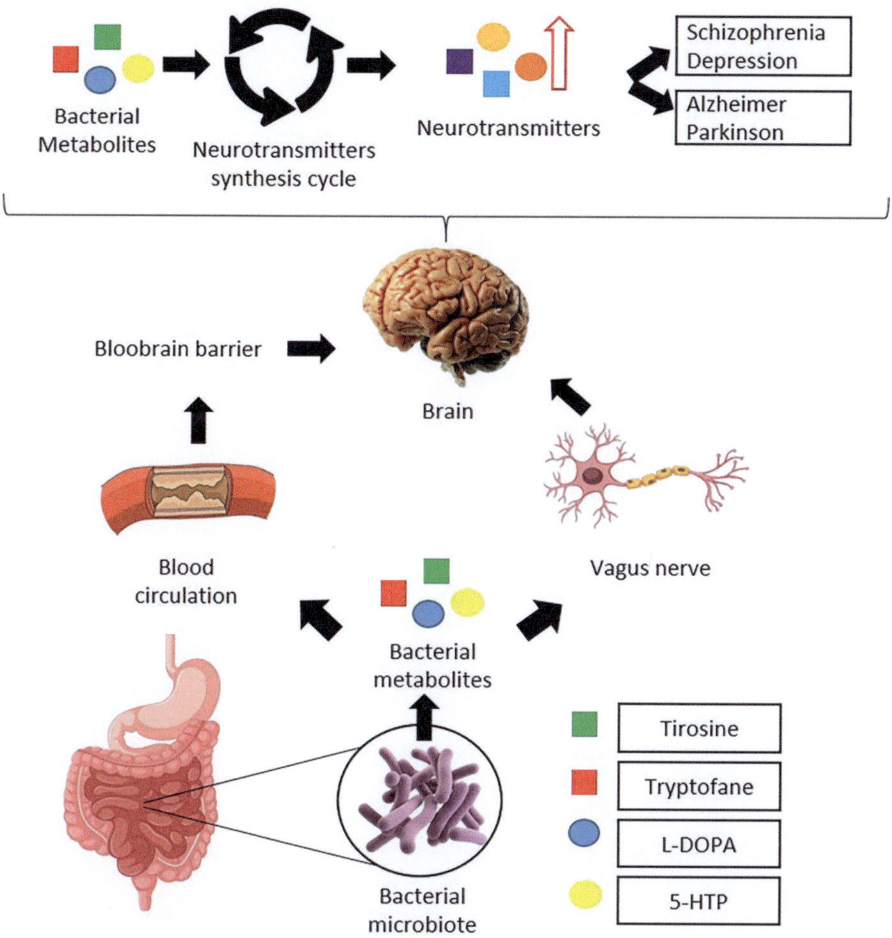

Fig. 3.1 Schematic representation of the microbiota-gut-brain axis and the pathway of bacterial metabolites to reach the brain

levels that leads to the development of diseases such as schizophrenia or autism and in cognitive disorders in Alzheimer's and Parkinson's disease. On the contrary, low levels of neurotransmitters in the brain may imply a deficiency in the synthesis of neurotransmitters or their intestinal precursors. The bacterial intestinal microbiota can modify neurotransmitter levels by modulating the amino acids tyrosine and tryptophan provided by the diet. On the other hand, the bacteria of the microbiota are capable of modifying the release of endocrine signals, which are produced by the enteroendocrine cells of the intestine in a physiological way. Certain types of precursors carried by bacteria act as signaling molecules for enteroendocrine cells, causing levels of neurotransmitters or intestinal peptides to be synthesized independently of the orders of the ANS. An important fact to highlight is that although neurotransmitters cannot cross the blood-brain barrier due to their macromolecular size, they can exert their actions on nerve endings in peripheral organs. In relation to the transport of sensory information, a type of neuroendocrine cells called neuropod cells (*neuropod cells)* can synapse with the vagus nerve via glutamate to transmit the sugar stimulus to the intestine. Intestinal motility may also be mediated by microbiota bacteria and serotonin-releasing enterochromaffin cells. Bacterial metabolites are detected by enterochromaffin cells causing the release of serotonin and with the consequent activation of enteric motor fibers and promoting gastrointestinal motility.

3.1.3 Blood-Brain Barrier

The blood-brain barrier is a structure at the cellular level that connects the blood capillaries in the brain with the nerve cells. It is characterized by being formed by blood capillaries wrapped by astrocytic feet that receive the molecules that circulate through the blood and act as a filter preventing harmful circulating molecules from accessing the neurons directly. Certain neurotransmitter precursor molecules, seen in the previous point, are capable of passing through, thus being able to access the neurons, which synthesize neurotransmitters. Increased permeability of the barrier increases the susceptibility for toxins and molecules produced by the microbiota to access the brain.

3.2 Neurodegenerative Diseases

Neurodegenerative diseases are a group of pathologies that affect the brain parenchyma, to a greater or lesser extent a specific structure, and peripheral nervous tissue. They are diseases characterized by progressive deterioration due to cellular and molecular alterations and environmental and dietary influence. They cause symptoms associated with disabling and dependent behavior of the patient, along with cognitive deficits. They are diseases that seriously affect the lives of patients and their families.

3.2.1 Alzheimer's Disease and Microbiota

3.2.1.1 Beta-Amyloid Deposits and Hyperphosphorylated Tau Protein

Alzheimer's disease (AD) is the most common progressive neurodegenerative disease in the elderly. The elderly demographic group mostly presents dementia due to Alzheimer's disease, which makes it the most prevalent type of dementia, accounting for 60–70% of dementia cases, according to the World Health Organization (WHO). The molecular bases of this pathology mainly affect the CNS. Neuronal affection in the brain is produced by the accumulation of two protein aggregates: extracellular neuritic plaques of beta-amyloid (derived from amyloid precursor protein or APP) and accumulation of hyperphosphorylated tau protein in the form of neurofibrils. The formation of these pathological aggregates is accompanied or is the cause or consequence of other neuronal metabolic alterations such as oxidative stress, microgliosis, deregulation of neuronal proteolysis, or neuroinflammation. In addition, external factors such as infections or brain damage from trauma can drive the progression of the pathology. In relation to dysbiosis, the disproportion by increase in the ratio of *Firmicutes/Bacteroidetes* populations causes intestinal accumulation of APP in early stages of Alzheimer's disease. Knowledge of the influence of the intestinal microbiota on neurodegenerative diseases has been obtained from studies carried out in germ-free mice and transgenic mice. One of the most important results was the finding of an increase in beta-amyloid at the CNS level in APP/PS1 mice, added to the impairment of learning and memory. In Alzheimer's disease mice, aberrant accumulations of beta-amyloid in myenteric neurons and activation of intestinal innate immunity were observed in a period prior to the onset of neuroinflammation. In a specific strain of transgenic AD model mice (Tg2576 mice), they present intestinal dysbiosis, intestinal barrier dysfunction, and vascular deposition of beta-amyloid prior to beta-amyloid deposition in the brain. In autopsies of brains of AD patients, the presence of beta-amyloid deposits at the intestinal level was detected. With respect to function, beta-amyloid proteins behave similarly to prion proteins: they are transmitted from neuron to neuron, generating the cellular lesions typical of Alzheimer's disease. This knowledge about the behavior of beta-amyloid molecules opens a new branch of research related to personalized nutrition and a therapeutic strategy to modify these pathological protein deposits.

3.2.1.2 Gut Microbiota Metabolites

The release of bacterial metabolites influences the accumulation of harmful proteins. The SCFAs (*short chain fatty acids* or short chain fatty acids) interfere with the protein-protein interaction through which normal physiological proteins but also beta-amyloid proteins are assembled. Another type of metabolite is the *microbial-derived metabolite trimethylamine* or TMAO. TMAOs cause cognitive impairment and pathological processes in AD by promoting the deposition of beta-amyloid by promoting the activation of beta-secretase enzymes and allowing access of activated platelets to the brain. TMAO synthesis drives platelet hyperactivation by stimulating the release of intracellular calcium ions from storage organelles. In this way, the synthesis of beta-amyloid in platelets is promoted so that they can enter the cerebral blood circulation (Fig. 3.2).

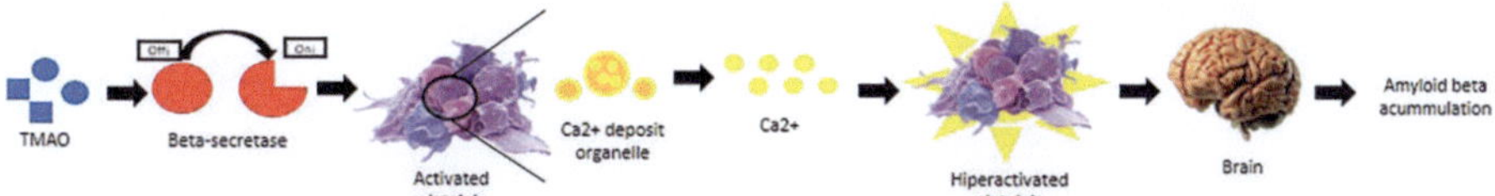

Fig. 3.2 Schematic representation of platelet hyperactivation mediated by TMAOs

The increase in circulating bacteria produces the synthesis of bile acids (BAs), which disturb the elimination routes of cholesterol, which accumulates and increases the synthesis of beta-amyloid. BAs increase the permeability of the BBB by interacting and destroying tight junctions (*tight junctions*) that stabilize the different components of the barrier. BAs and peripheral circulating cholesterol can enter the CNS, where cholesterol binds to APP and facilitates its deposit in the phospholipid layers, specifically in membrane locations known as lipid *rafts*, in which the formation of beta-amyloid takes place. The brain condition due to cholesterol accumulation is induced by the interaction between BAs and farnesoid (farnesoid *X receptor*), which induces downregulation of the expression of the enzyme CYP46A, which metabolizes cholesterol.

Certain metabolites released by bacteria exert a mechanism of molecular mimicry (*molecular mimicry*). Bacterial amyloids can act as prion proteins to alter and aggregate with amyloids in the patient's body. Table 3.1 shows bacterial amyloids with this property.

3.2.1.3 Microglia and Microbiota in Alzheimer's Disease

Pathological activation of microglia due to dysbiosis is associated with Alzheimer's disease. Under physiological conditions, the phagocytic capacity of microglia is essential for the elimination of soluble beta-amyloid molecules and fibrillar deposits. Activated microglia in the vicinity of amyloid deposits prevent the formation of compact aggregates and new toxic beta-amyloid plaques, as well as minimizing damage to adjacent neuropodia. The microbiota appears to be necessary for the maturation of microglia and their homeostasis. Defects are observed in microglia with respect to cell proportions, immature phenotypes, and downregulation of the expression of microglia maturation genes in germ-free mice and SPF mice (*specific-pathogen-free*). Germ-free mice show an improvement in microglia with the implementation of SCFAs or transfusion of healthy microbiota. Microglia from SPF mice show deficits in SCFA receptor 2, and their phenotype is identical to that of germ-free mice. It was concluded that microglia are very sensitive to changes in the intestinal microbiota community and its metabolites.

Table 3.1 It shows the most common amyloids that perform molecular mimicry and the bacteria species that produce them

Bacteria species	Produced amyloid
Escherichia coli	Curly amyloid
Pseudomonas fluorescens	FapC
Staphylococcus aureus	Phenol-soluble modulins
Streptomyces coelicolor	*Chaplins*
Klebsiella pneumonia	MccE492

3.2.2 Parkinson's Disease and Microbiota

3.2.2.1 Gut Microbiota in Parkinson's Disease

Parkinson's disease is a degenerative disease caused by progressive loss of dopaminergic neurons and accumulation of alpha-synuclein in the substantia nigra and striatum in the brainstem. The decrease in dopaminergic neurons causes the characteristic motor symptoms of the pathology: tremors, bradykinesia, and postural instability. Patients often present with other non-motor symptoms such as behavioral changes, sleep disorders, and gastrointestinal dysfunction. Although motor symptoms are mostly associated with Parkinson's disease, non-motor symptoms play a dominant role in the clinical manifestations. Eighty percent of patients present severe gastrointestinal symptoms such as constipation, nausea, and vomiting, which has prompted research to try to find a relationship between the pathogenesis of the disease and dysbiosis.

In recent studies, the intestinal microbiotas of Parkinson's patients were compared with healthy subjects, in which significant differences were found in the types of bacterial populations and their changes as the stages of the disease progressed. The importance of the bacterial species that increase in Parkinson's patients is related to the decrease in the mucus layer that covers the intestinal epithelium and the functionality of dopaminergic neurons. The decrease in *Prevotellaceae* species, together with *Lachnospiraceae*, affects intestinal protection and the normal production of SCFAs through fermentation. The *Prevotellaceae* species protects against neurodegeneration due to mucin synthesis and ghrelin secretion. The loss of *Prevotellaceae* bacteria causes reduced levels of intestinal mucus and the production of SCFAs, worsening the patient's intestinal permeability and increasing the risk of local inflammation. Ghrelin is a stomach hormone that promotes feelings of appetite and protects the normal dopaminergic function of the substantia nigra by controlling mitochondrial respiration and the synthesis of reactive oxygen species. In the microbiota of Parkinson's disease patients, an increase in *Lactobacillaceae* species is observed, added to the aforementioned decrease in *Prevotellaceae*, thus leading to a decrease in ghrelin secretion and deterioration of dopaminergic function. In MPTP (1-methyl-4-phenyl-1,2,3,6-tetrahydropyridine) mouse models, ghrelin showed a protective effect on dopaminergic neurons by inhibiting the accumulation of a-synuclein, promoting autophagy and apoptosis mediated by the endoplasmic reticulum. In a clinical study, the total and active levels of ghrelin were measured in a group of patients. It is of great interest that patients with Parkinson's disease have decreased levels and demonstrate the usefulness of the study of plasma ghrelin levels as a diagnostic biomarker and treatment of Parkinson's disease (Fig. 3.3).

3.2.2.2 Nasal Microbiota in Parkinson's Disease

Some studies have suggested that there is no significant difference in the microbiota pool in the nasal cavity of patients with Parkinson's disease but that the microbiota shows great variability between different individuals. There is a great correlation

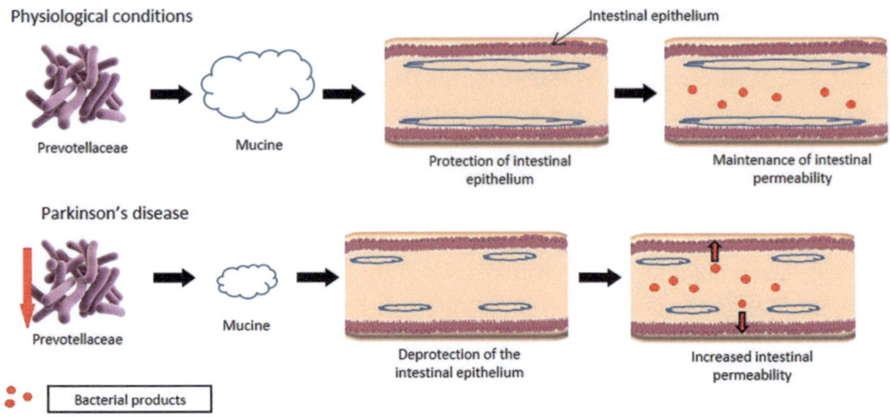

Fig. 3.3 Schematic representation of the protective effect of *Prevotellaceae* bacteria. When the population decreases, there is a lower concentration of mucin that coats the intestinal epithelium which favors the contact of toxins present in the lumen or PAMPs of bacteria of the microbiota

between alterations of the specific oral microbiota in taxonomy and functionality in Parkinson's disease patients.

3.2.2.3 Inflammation of the Enteric System, Microbiota, and Parkinson's Disease

There is a theory that suggests that Parkinson's disease is initiated by a process of intestinal inflammation. Intestinal inflammation is related to the microbiota because the different populations that make it up are located on the intestinal mucosa and interfere with it. The intestinal mucosa is a monolayer of epithelial tissue (simple cylindrical epithelial tissue with mucus-producing cells) that is located on the luminal side of the intestine (it presents variations depending on the section of the small intestine and with respect to the large intestine). The intestinal mucosa protects the intestine and peripheral organs by preventing microbiota bacteria from accessing the blood capillaries located in the submucosal layer. The epithelial cells of the intestinal mucosa and the microbiota are in a state of constant interaction: epithelial cells regulate the diversity and function of the microbiota; and the microbiota is crucial for the growth of epithelial cells. Parkinson's disease patients present inflammation in colonic tissues and elevation of inflammatory cytokines and chemokines (TNF, IL-1β, IL-17, IL-6, interferon gamma, or IFN-γ) and ECG reactive factor for the activation of proliferation and inflammation. At a clinical level, high levels of markers of intestinal inflammation (calprotectin) and intestinal barrier dysfunction (zunolin) were found, which argues in favor of the proposed hypothesis. Microbiota bacteria and their metabolites are involved in the pathophysiology of Parkinson's disease due to their promoting effects on intestinal inflammation and activation of the immune system. The following species of bacteria have been found related to Parkinson's disease (Table 3.2).

Table 3.2 Bacteria species related to the development of Parkinson's disease

Location	Microbiota bacteria species	Status of bacterial population levels	Effect they cause
Mucosa intestinal	Ralstonia	Abundant	Proinflamatorio
Parkinson's disease stool samples	Akkermansia Oscillospira Bacteroides	Increased	Proinflamatorio

Table 3.3 Subtypes of TLR and their known function in Parkinson's disease

TLR type	Expression zone	Receiver function
TLR2	↓ Human colon enteric neurons glial cells muscle cells of the intestinal wall	Deficiency of this receptor means the reduction of neurons and glial cells strong colonic inflammation
TLR3	Human small intestine and colon	–
TLR4	↓ Human colon	–
TLR5	↑ Human colon	–

Some of the bacterial species of the intestinal microbiota can interfere with the systemic inflammatory response. The *Bacteroides* population is associated with high plasma levels of TNF, and *Verrucomicrobiaceae* with plasma levels of IFN-γ. In Parkinson's disease patients, the *Roseburia* population is decreased and produces deregulations in the function of the immune system. *Roseburia* bacteria can promote the expression of immune genes such as antimicrobial peptide genes, intestinal barrier maintenance genes, and receptor-like genes. *Toll-like receptor 5* or TLR5 promotes the reduction of inflammation in addition to a correct function of the intestinal barrier. *Roseburia* species promote immune system homeostasis by inhibiting NF-kB. High expression of TLR can increase the permeability of the intestinal epithelial barrier and the susceptibility to colonic inflammation (Table 3.3).

3.2.2.4 Functions and Infiltration of Immune Cells in Brain with Parkinson's Disease

One of the components that interact directly with the microbiota, especially the intestinal microbiota, are the different components of the immune system. Studies carried out in Parkinson's disease patients and in transgenic mouse models of this disease and other types of models have shown the relationship between altered immunity and the appearance of the neurodegenerative disease. One of the cells analyzed in Parkinson's disease patients are peripheral monocytes, offering insight into the role of peripheral cells in neuroinflammation. In mouse models of Parkinson's disease, overexpression of alpha-synuclein facilitates the entry of proinflammatory C–C chemokine receptor type 2-positive monocytes into the CNS. In contrast, deletion of the CCR2 receptor prevents monocyte infiltration, alpha-synuclein-mediated inflammation, and dopaminergic neuron death. Other studies focused on the role of cytotoxic (CD8+) and helper (CD3+/CD4+) T lymphocytes in their ability to infiltrate the brain and generate disease. T cell infiltrates were found in post-mortem midbrain sections of Parkinson's disease patients, and, to verify their lethality, pluripotent human stem cells derived from midbrain neurons were exposed to T lymphocytes, which generated interleukin-mediated neuronal death (IL)-17 and NF-kB. On the other hand, the infiltration of cytotoxic T lymphocytes occurs prior to the accumulation of alpha-synuclein and neuronal death. In alpha-synuclein transgenic mouse models, infiltration of T helper cells is increased in the vicinity of astrocytes and microglia, with notable glial activation and expression of tumor necrosis factor (TNF) genes. It was determined that the infiltration of peripheral lymphocytes promotes the activation of resident immune cells in the brain.

3.2.3 Multiple Sclerosis and Microbiota

Multiple sclerosis (MS) is an autoimmune disease in which lymphocytes and multinucleated cells infiltrate the cerebral cortex and directly attack oligodendrocytes. Oligodendrocytes are nerve cells that constitute the myelin sheaths in neuronal axons in the CNS. The destruction of these cells causes the nervous impulse to be ineffective, which manifests clinically as functional deterioration of the patient, whether in the control of their physiological needs, such as motility and the perception of sensations. It is a progressive disease that occurs in patients between 20 and 40 years of age and/or with a history of Epstein-Barr virus infection or vitamin D deficiency. Regarding the condition between sexes, a ratio of 2:1 is established for women and 3:1, debuting at earlier ages in women and later in men, and for these with a faster progression and greater severity. Multiple sclerosis is characterized by the appearance of outbreaks, in which the patient suffers the symptoms of neuronal deterioration, interspersed by recurrent stages. It should be noted that the symptoms mentioned depend on the subtype of multiple sclerosis (Table 3.4).

3.2.3.1 Etiology of Multiple Sclerosis in Relation to the TLR2 Receptor, the Microbiota, and the Hygiene Hypothesis

Researcher Nicholas J. Wasko, along with Frank Nichols and Robert B. Clark, led the project *Multiple Sclerosis, the Microbiome, TLR2 and the Hygiene Hypothesis*, which provided a new perspective on the cause and risk factors of this disease. Over

Table 3.4 Subtypes of multiple sclerosis and clinical manifestations

Multiple sclerosis subtype	Clinical manifestations of outbreaks and recurrences
Relapsing-remitting multiple sclerosis (RRMS)	Outbreaks with exacerbations followed by periods of remission of symptoms. It can evolve to SPMS
Secondary progressive multiple sclerosis (SPMS)	It is the most serious subtype because neuronal deterioration occurs in each new outbreak without improvement despite treatment
Primary progressive multiple sclerosis (PPMS)	There are no periods of remission, but rather it is established in a stabilized phase of symptoms that entails gradual worsening
Progressive with exacerbations	It is a progressive form with sudden worsening and no remissions. It is the rarest subtype

the last decade, they carried out laboratory tests that revealed a crucial connection between multiple sclerosis, the hygiene hypothesis, and the microbiota through the TLR2 receptor.

A unique family of bacterial lipopeptides known as "serine lipids" has been identified, originating from *Bacteroides* species present in the oral and gastrointestinal tract. These lipopeptides are recognized by immune system cells through the TLR2 receptor. In particular, members of the Lipid 654 family, which have structural differences from human lipids, have been found in blood samples from both healthy individuals and those suffering from multiple sclerosis. It is suggested that chronic stimulation of TLR2 by microbiota-derived PAMPs (Pathogen-Associated Molecular Patterns) coexists in the blood circulation along with normal mammalian lipids. Surprisingly, L654 concentration levels were in the lower ranges compared to healthy individuals. This finding is puzzling, since multiple sclerosis is an autoimmune disease associated with inflammation of the central nervous system, which could have suggested higher levels in people with this condition. However, this paradox is explained by the dual function of the TLR2 receptor, which can both activate proinflammatory pathways and also induce a state of TL2 tolerance. This state of normal "tolerance" of TLR2 is not sufficient to completely inhibit TLR2 signaling. Instead, it acts as a microbiome-driven regulator, attenuating or "fine-tuning" the magnitude of systemic TLR2 responses without completely inhibiting them. This microbiome-driven regulation of TLR2 responsiveness has evolved to protect the host from overreacting to endogenous TLR2 stimulants, such as DAMPs, while preserving the ability to respond appropriately and proinflammatorily to the strong signals and high concentrations of TLR2 PAMPs present during an infection. In multiple sclerosis patients, microbiome does not release normal levels of TLR2 PAMPS into the blood, and in the subsequent TLR2 responses are not induced to a correct tolerance, and it is insufficient to completely inhibit TLR2 signaling. The poor TLR2 tolerance induction enhances TLR2 responses that promote overexpression of DAMPs (that means the activation of auto-reactivity) and defective remyelination.

The activation of autoreactive T and B lymphocytes, especially CD4+ lymphocytes, in peripheral lymph nodes and their differentiation promotes the activation cascade of autoimmune cells that damage the CNS. Regulatory T lymphocytes suffer alterations in which they lose their ability to suppress the autoreactive response, triggering the uncontrolled activation of T helper lymphocytes of the Th1, Th17, and Th22 type, which circulate through the blood to the CNS. Upon crossing the blood-brain barrier, they behave as antigen-presenting cells (APC) and recognize myelin components as antigens, initiating the release of cytokines and chemokines that promote inflammation and attraction of more autoreactive cells circulating in the blood. Upon receiving stimuli from the immune response in the CNS, mature B lymphocytes and plasma cells synthesize antibodies that feed back on the activation of TCD4+ lymphocytes and maintain and increase the inflammatory process at the CNS level. The inflammatory process activates microglia cells that attack the myelin sheaths. At the intracellular level, TLR2-mediated inflammation involves the activation of the MyD88 and TRIF pathways. MyD88 attracts the TRAF6, IRAK, and

NF-kB proteins that translocate to the cell nucleus and activate the expression of genes that encode TNF-α and COX-2. These proteins are responsible for generating inflammation at the central nervous system (CNS), among others (Fig. 3.4).

The Hygiene Theory postulates that due to excessive cleaning of the most frequent environment in which human beings live, it causes the immaturity of the immune system. The term "cleanliness" in this context mainly refers to the low presence of common microorganisms and microorganism-derived molecules (pathogen-associated molecular patterns or "PAMPs"). The deficiency of PAMPs in daily activities is detrimental to the development of immune cell responses and is established as one of the factors for the development of autoimmune diseases such as asthma and allergic diseases. Over-reactive and exaggerated immune responses are the consequence of chronic exposure to such a low presence of PAMP. Epidemiological studies in Europe ensure protection against asthma and allergies in children raised on traditional farms with high exposure to microorganisms and animals (Table 3.5).

3.2.3.2 Innovation in Diagnostic Methods with Biomarkers

Due to the characteristics of the disease (degenerative damage to the brain), the methodology for diagnosis is usually using imaging tests. To date, there are no serological tests approved for the reliable diagnosis of the disease, such as the finding of rheumatoid factor and cyclic citrullinated peptide for the diagnosis of rheumatoid arthritis. The most reliable and routine imaging test as a diagnostic tool for MS is

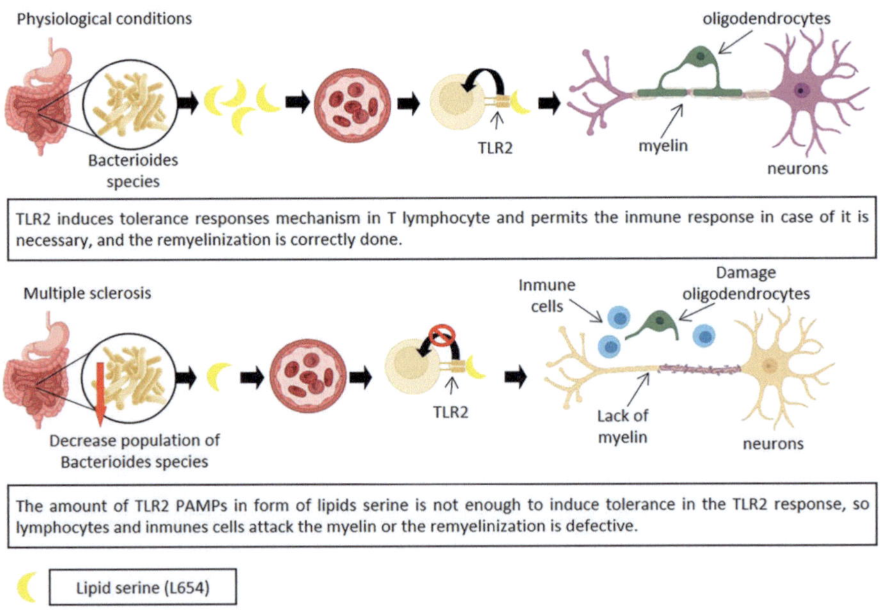

Fig. 3.4 Schematic representation of the effect of inefficient TLR2 induction and myelin sheath deterioration

Table 3.5 Comparison of patterns of bacterial populations and their status in multiple sclerosis patients and control groups

Stade of populations	MS patients	Control group
↑	- *Methanobrevibacter.* - *Akkermansia.* - *Prevotella* in treated patients. - *Sutterella* in treated patients. - *Pseudomonas.* - *Mycoplana.* - *Haemophilus.* - *Blautia.* - *Dorea.*	↑ *Parabacteroides* ↑ *Adlercreutzia* ↑ *Prevotella*
↓	- *Butyricimonas.* - *Sarcina* in treated patients.	

magnetic resonance imaging (MRI), in which specialists can find signs of gray and white matter destruction. The lesions are indicative of inflammation coupled with neuroaxonal damage and demyelination, which are known as demyelination plaques. Despite the importance of this imaging test, it has a series of limitations. Routine MRI lacks high sensitivity and specificity for the detection of neurodegeneration. It measures the thinness of the individual's cortex, which is subject to interpersonal variations that can be modified by other factors such as age. Another common way to diagnose MS is the analysis of cerebrospinal fluid (CSF). It is more preferable than blood test as it reflects CNS inflammation and shows higher sensitivity compared to MRI in MS patients with low-grade activity. In the analysis of CSF fluid, two molecules are considered: light chain neurofilaments (cNfL) and the immunoglobulin (Ig) G index, which is usually found in high concentrations. At the serum level, sNfL is studied, which is usually elevated in MS patients prior to the appearance of symptoms.

3.3 Brain Diseases and Microbiota

The brain diseases that will be treated in this chapter are psychiatric disorders in which behavior, the management of emotions, and the perception of reality are affected. There is no deterioration of the brain parenchyma as such, but rather imbalances in the neurotransmitters and their normal levels.

3.3.1 Psychiatric Illnesses and Cognitive Disorders

3.3.1.1 Factors that Alter the Microbiota and Mental Illnesses

Periods of stress in humans have been shown to cause alterations in alpha-diversity (number and distribution of the microbiota) and beta-diversity (compositional differences). As a consequence, a radical decrease in the number of *Lactobacillus* and *Bifidobacterium* is observed; in mice, there is an increase in the *Clostridium* species and, due to the secretion of catecholamines (adrenaline and norepinephrine), also in the number of pathogenic and non-pathogenic *Escherichia coli* bacteria. Long-term stress and suffering at an early age are related to the development of mental disorders and diseases, such as depression and anxiety. It initiates in the hypothalamic-pituitary-adrenal (HPA) axis, where large concentrations of corticotropin-releasing hormone (CRH) are secreted from the hypothalamus, and has a synergistic action with arginine vasopressin (AVP). CRH reaches the pituitary gland or adenohypophysis where it activates the release of adrenocorticotropic hormone (ACTH), which reaches the adrenal glands and promotes the secretion of cortisol. The hormone cortisol is known as "the stress hormone." In periods of continued stress, this axis remains active and with a high concentration of cortisol in plasma. Excess cortisol shows signs of strong psychological effects of anxiety, depression, sleep and eating dysregulations, and physical changes (decreased immune function, weight gain, hair loss). In recent studies it has been observed that in affective disorders, along with alterations in the field of neurotransmitters and neurohormones, there are also structural changes in the central nervous system. These affect structures of the hippocampus and the prefrontal cortex and are based on the reduction in the number of cells and the weakening of neurogenesis and neuronal plasticity processes.

Affected by stress and influenced by the microbiota, the circadian rhythm is one of the systems that can contribute to the appearance of psychiatric diseases. The circadian rhythm is an intrinsic rhythm in the body that manages different processes. The circadian clock system is located in the suprachiasmatic nucleus of the hypothalamus (CNS) and in small areas of tissues of peripheral organs such as the intestine, pancreas, heart, liver, skeletal muscles, and kidneys. The intestinal microbiota presents fluctuations during the day that can be affected by external factors such as work shift, jetlag, sleep, diet, or the aforementioned stress. In studies to analyze the imprint of stress on the microbiota, they demonstrated that exposure to social stress caused a decrease in the population of *Lactobacillus*, which exerts immunomodulatory functions in the colon. Some researchers pointed out that psychiatric and metabolic disorders are associated with disturbances in the circadian clock at the brain and peripheral level, specifically in the intestine, which can result in dysbiosis, bacterial translocations, and the increased risk of developing inflammation in metabolic diseases. At the cellular and molecular level, human circadian behavior has been shown to be controlled by "clock genes" and that the microbiota itself can modify the circadian clock of peripheral organs, such as the intestine and reprogramming the liver. Although the mechanisms for synchronization are not completely known, it is known from research that the circadian system regulates the microbiota through signals from bacterial clocks (*bacterial clocks*). In the intestine, amounts of melatonin were found, the sleep-wake regulatory hormone that was secreted on *site* and that favors the growth of Enterobacter aerogenes (a commensal bacteria of the human digestive tract). The microbiota participates in the reprogramming and homeostasis of the hepatic circadian clock through the peroxisome *proliferator-activated receptor-γ* (PPARγ) transcriptional, which modifies gene expression related to circadian activity.

3.3.1.2 Major Depressive Disorder

Major depressive disorder (*major depression disorder* or MDD) is a common mental disorder state, characterized by feelings of sadness and apathy lasting at least 2 weeks. It is the result of social events, psychological alterations, and biological factors (changes in the family, chronic diseases, addictions). Suicide is one of the main causes of death in patients with major depression. Recent research has demonstrated the relationship of this mental disorder with components of the intestinal microbiota, such as *Alistipes* genus and *Oscillibacter* species. *Alistipes* genus levels are associated with inflammation; and *Oscillibacter*, which produces valeric acid (*valeric acid*), is found at high concentrations in patients with major depression. In studies with mouse models, microbiota dysbiosis was associated with increased intestinal permeability and systemic inflammation. Studying mouse models of reduced endogenous melatonin (*endogenous melatonin reduction* or EMR), the composition of the intestinal microbiota was modified by the reduction of *Bacteroidetes*, the alteration of the *Firmicutes*/*Bacteroidetes* ratio, and the growth of *Lactobacillus*. Along with these changes, increased intestinal permeability and systemic inflammation were observed in EMR mice. In a study carried out on women with MDD to analyze the composition of their microbiota by determining the content of SCFAs, a difference was observed in the levels of acids secreted by bacteria. Of patients diagnosed with depression, 40.52%, compared to healthy patients, showed a lower level of propionic acid (*propionic acid*) and a higher isocaproic acid content (*isocaproic acid*). Despite these results, it was not possible to conclude the concentrations of SCFAs that determine an MDD phenotype. In animal models, the connection between the intestinal microbiota, behavior, and personality was found. In individuals of Mongolian gerbils (*Meriones clawed*) underwent gut microbiota transplants to study behavioral change. Gerbils with a shy disposition that received a microbiota transplant from individuals with bold behavior subsequently exhibited behavior similar to that of the individual from whom they received the microbiota transplant.

3.4 Precision Medicine and Microbiota

Precision medicine represents an innovative way to approach the prevention, diagnosis, treatment, and prognosis of diseases. Although it is based on the principles of traditional medicine, it is enriched with the use of advanced technologies and the latest scientific advances, especially in the fields of genetics and immunology, with a molecular approach. One of the prominent fields in precision medicine is the study of the microbiota, given that knowledge of its functions and its application in the treatment and cure of diseases constitutes an essential aspect of this discipline. In the context of neurodegenerative diseases such as Alzheimer's, Parkinson's, and amyotrophic lateral sclerosis (ALS), precision medicine seeks to understand the genetic and molecular differences between patients to develop specific and effective treatments. In the search for innovative therapeutic approaches, various strategies involving modulation of the microbiota are being investigated. These include the use of probiotics, which are beneficial microorganisms that can help restore a healthy balance to the gut microbiota. In addition, prebiotics, which are substances that promote the growth of beneficial microorganisms, are also being studied in this context. Additionally, specific diets designed to promote a healthy microbiota are being viewed as a promising approach.

Suggested Readings

1. Mou Y, Du Y, Zhou L, Yue J, Hu X, Liu Y, et al. Gut microbiota interact with the brain through systemic chronic inflammation: implications on neuroinflammation, neurodegeneration, and aging. Front Immunol. 2022;13:796288. https://pubmed.ncbi.nlm.nih.gov/35464431/
2. Góralczyk-Bińkowska A, Szmajda-Krygier D, Kozłowska E. The microbiota–gut–brain axis in psychiatric disorders. Int J Mol Sci. 2022;23(19):11245. https://doi.org/10.3390/ijms231911245.
3. Morais LH, Schreiber HL IV, Mazmanian SK. The gut microbiota–brain axis in behaviour and brain disorders. Nat Rev Microbiol. 2021;19(4):241–55. https://pubmed.ncbi.nlm.nih.gov/33093662/
4. Chen Y, Xu J, Chen Y. Regulation of neurotransmitters by the gut microbiota and effects on cognition in neurological disorders. Nutrients. 2021;13(6):2099. https://doi.org/10.3390/nu13062099.
5. Wang Q, Luo Y, Ray Chaudhuri K, Reynolds R, Tan E-K, Pettersson S. The role of gut dysbiosis in Parkinson's disease: mechanistic insights and therapeutic options. Brain. 2021;144(9):2571–93. https://pubmed.ncbi.nlm.nih.gov/33856024/
6. Cersosimo MG, Raina GB, Pecci C, Pellene A, Calandra CR, Gutiérrez C, et al. Gastrointestinal manifestations in Parkinson's disease: prevalence and occurrence before motor symptoms. J Neurol. 2013;260(5):1332–8. https://pubmed.ncbi.nlm.nih.gov/23263478/
7. Yang D, Zhao D, Ali Shah SZ, Wu W, Lai M, Zhang X, et al. The role of the gut microbiota in the pathogenesis of Parkinson's disease. Front Neurol. 2019;10:1155. https://pubmed.ncbi.nlm.nih.gov/31781020/
8. Heiss CN, Olofsson LE. The role of the gut microbiota in development, function and disorders of the central nervous system and the enteric nervous system. J Neuroendocrinol. 2019;31(5):e12684. https://pubmed.ncbi.nlm.nih.gov/30614568/
9. Tremlett H, Bauer KC, Appel-Cresswell S, Finlay BB, Waubant E. The gut microbiome in human neurological disease: a review: gut microbiome. Ann Neurol. 2017;81(3):369–82. https://doi.org/10.1002/ana.24901.
10. Li C, Cui L, Yang Y, Miao J, Zhao X, Zhang J, et al. Gut microbiota differs between Parkinson's disease patients and healthy controls in Northeast China. Front Mol Neurosci. 2019;12:171. https://doi.org/10.3389/fnmol.2019.00171.
11. Heneka MT, Carson MJ, Khoury JE, Landreth GE, Brosseron F, Feinstein DL, et al. Neuroinflammation in Alzheimer's disease. Lancet Neurol. 2015;14(4):388–405. https://doi.org/10.1016/s1474-4422(15)70016-5.
12. Long-Smith C, O'Riordan KJ, Clarke G, Stanton C, Dinan TG, Cryan JF. Microbiota-gut-brain axis: new therapeutic opportunities. Annu Rev Pharmacol Toxicol. 2020;60(1):477–502. https://doi.org/10.1146/annurev-pharmtox-010919-023628.
13. Kim M-S, Kim Y, Choi H, Kim W, Park S, Lee D, et al. Transfer of a healthy microbiota reduces amyloid and tau pathology in an Alzheimer's disease animal model. Gut. 2020;69(2):283–94. https://doi.org/10.1136/gutjnl-2018-317431.
14. An LJ, Gibson DL, Klegeris A. Unhealthy gut, unhealthy brain: the role of the intestinal microbiota in neurodegenerative diseases. Neurochem Int. 2018;120:149–63.
15. Hooper LV, Littman DR, Macpherson AJ. Interactions between the microbiota and the immune system. Science. 2012;336(6086):1268–73. https://doi.org/10.1126/science.1223490.

16. Fung TC, Olson CA, Hsiao EY. Interactions between the microbiota, immune and nervous systems in health and disease. Nat Neurosci. 2017;20(2):145–55. https://doi.org/10.1038/nn.4476.
17. Du L, Zhang Y, Chen Y, Zhu J, Yang Y, Zhang H-L. Role of microglia in neurological disorders and their potentials as a therapeutic target. Mol Neurobiol. 2017;54(10):7567–84. https://doi.org/10.1007/s12035-016-0245-0.
18. Gulas E, Wysiadecki G, Strzelecki D, Gawlik-Kotelnicka O, Polguj M. Can microbiology affect psychiatrists? A link between gut microbiota and psychiatric disorders. Psychiatr Pol. 2018;52(6):1023–39. https://doi.org/10.12740/pp/onlinefirst/81103.
19. Fond G, Boukouaci W, Chevalier G, Regnault A, Eberl G, Hamdani N, et al. The "psychomicrobiotic": targeting microbiota in major psychiatric disorders: a systematic review. Pathol Biol (Paris). 2015;63(1):35–42. https://doi.org/10.1016/j.patbio.2014.10.003.
20. Cryan JF, Dinan TG. Mind-altering microorganisms: the impact of the gut microbiota on brain and behaviour. Nat Rev Neurosci. 2012;13(10):701–12. https://www.nature.com/articles/nrn3346
21. Yang J, Hamade M, Wu Q, Wang Q, Axtell R, Giri S, et al. Current and future biomarkers in multiple sclerosis. Int J Mol Sci. 2022;23(11):5877. https://doi.org/10.3390/ijms23115877.
22. Wasko NJ, Nichols F, Clark RB. Multiple sclerosis, the microbiome, TLR2, and the hygiene hypothesis. Autoimmun Rev. 2020;19(1):102430. https://doi.org/10.1016/j.autrev.2019.102430.
23. Bach J-F. The hygiene hypothesis in autoimmunity: the role of pathogens and commensals. Nat Rev Immunol. 2018;18(2):105–20. https://doi.org/10.1038/nri.2017.111.
24. Van Schependom J, Dhooghe MB, Cleynhens K, Dhooge M, Haelewyck MC, De Keyser J, Nagels G. The symbol digit modalities test as sentinel test for cognitive impairment in multiple sclerosis. Eur J Neurol. 2014;21(9):1219–25. e71-2
25. Rocca MA, Battaglini M, Benedict RHB, De Stefano N, Geurts JJG, Henry RG, et al. Brain MRI atrophy quantification in MS: from methods to clinical application. Neurology. 2017;88(4):403–13. https://doi.org/10.1212/WNL.0000000000003542.

Microbiota and Diseases Associated with the Digestive System

4

Andrea Martín-Rivas

4.1 Introduction

Over the past few years, a great deal of research and clinical work has been carried out to deepen our understanding of the intestinal microbiota and its function, development and influence on the pathogenesis of certain diseases [1].

The term microflora or microbiota refers to a group of microorganisms that gather in a specific ecological niche. The gut microbiota includes native gut microorganisms that live permanently in the gut and various microorganisms that transit the gut for short periods of time. Native gut bacteria are acquired at birth and in the first year of life, while transient bacteria are acquired through beverages, food, etc. [2]. The human gut microbiome consists of 100 trillion bacteria of 500–1000 different species [3, 4]. The stomach and duodenum contain a small number of microorganisms that are attached to or move through the mucosa. Acid, bile and pancreatic secretions remove most of the ingested microorganisms, and motor-driven activity prevents continued colonisation of the lumen. The number of bacteria in the jejunum and ileum gradually increases, and gram-negative aerobic bacteria and some obligate anaerobic bacteria predominate. In comparison, the large intestine is densely populated with anaerobic microorganisms. The large intestine has been used to characterise non-culturable bacteria, and currently unknown strains are being identified [5, 6].

Mammals reared in strict sterile conditions do not acquire their natural flora and develop abnormally. There are defects of the digestive system with atrophy of the intestinal walls and changes in motility, reduced metabolism with generalised weight loss, decreased cardiac function, low blood flow, low body temperature and increased blood cholesterol, as well as an immature immune system with low levels of immunoglobulins and an atrophied lymphatic system. Therefore, the presence of

A. Martín-Rivas (✉)
Department of Biomedicine, Universidad Alfonso X, Madrid, Spain

J. Ruiz-Tovar (ed.), *Dysbiosis*, https://doi.org/10.1007/978-3-031-65650-7_4

certain bacteria in the intestinal flora is important for proper nutrition and physical development, as well as for maintaining immunity. Intestinal homeostasis is very important for absorbing energy from food and protecting it from pathogens [7, 8].

The relationship between the host and its flora is one of symbiosis (one species benefits without causing harm to the others). The host provides a habitat and nutrients for the microorganisms, and the microbiome contributes to the physiology of the host [7].

4.1.1 Functions of the Microbiota

Gut colonisation studies have identified three main activities of the gut microbiota:

- Nutritional and metabolic functions resulting from the biochemical activities of the flora, including energy recovery, production of short-chain fatty acids and a beneficial effect on the absorption of vitamins, calcium and iron in the colon [2].
- Protective functions preventing the entry of infectious agents or overgrowth of native species with pathogenic potential [2].
- Trophic functions on the proliferation and differentiation of the intestinal epithelium and development and regulation of the immune system [2].

4.1.1.1 Metabolic Functions

The gut flora metabolises undigestible food substrates or residues, endogenous mucus and cellular debris. The genetic diversity of the microbial community provides resources for the host and many other enzymes and biochemical pathways [9].

Fermentation of non-host-digestible carbohydrates occurs mainly in the cecum and right colon. This provides an important source of energy for bacterial growth and produces short-chain fatty acids that can be absorbed by the host. This means that energy from food is transformed and promotes the absorption of ions (Ca, Mg, Fe) in the cecum. Metabolic functions also include the synthesis of vitamins (K, B12, biotin, folic acid and pantothenic acid) and amino acids from ammonia or urea [10]. Anaerobic metabolism (breakdown) of peptides and proteins occurs in the more distal parts of the colon and is a source of short-chain fatty acids but also produces a variety of potentially toxic substances such as ammonia, amines, thiols, phenols and indoles [11, 12].

4.1.1.2 Protective Functions

The protective functions of the microbiota include a barrier effect of bacteria occupying an ecological niche or space, preventing the translocation of foreign bacteria into the ecosystem. In addition, the local microbiota prevents overgrowth of opportunistic bacteria present in the gut, but with limited reproduction. The balance between local bacterial species confers stability to the whole. The proliferation inhibitory effect depends on the ability of bacteria to secrete antimicrobial substances and on the competition between bacteria for system resources such as nutrients or ecological space [13, 14].

4.1.1.3 Trophic Functions

Intestinal bacteria can control the proliferation and differentiation of epithelial cells [15]. In colony niches of animals cultured under strictly sterile conditions, there was a reduction in the rate of epithelial cell turnover compared to animals with a normal microbiota. Epithelial cell differentiation is strongly influenced by interactions with the microorganisms that inhabit them, as demonstrated by the expression of various genes in animals associated with bacterial strains [7].

Bacteria also play an important role in the development of the immune system. In animals reared under strict aseptic conditions, lymphocyte concentrations in the small intestinal mucosa are low, the structure of lymphoid follicles is lost, and circulating immunoglobulin concentrations are abnormally low, whereas in animals with a normal microbiota, these parameters are not altered [16, 17].

4.1.2 Intestinal Microbiota and the Immune System

The gastrointestinal tract is a very sensitive interface for contact and communication between the individual and the external environment. To achieve homeostasis, the individual must distinguish between pathogens on the one hand and commensal microorganisms in symbiosis with the host on the other hand. In the first case, it must possess adequate defence elements, and in the second case, the host must be able to tolerate them. The interactions between microorganisms, epithelium and lymphoid tissue in the gut are very diverse and therefore constantly regenerate local and systemic immune mechanisms, adapting to the microbiological environment [18].

The epithelial cell plays a pivotal role in the immune system, being in the first line of defence and in direct contact with the intestinal lumen. Its location is crucial for the initial recognition of foreign substances and for the transmission of signals to immunocompetent cells in the underlying tissue. Activation of defence mechanisms depends primarily on the rapid recognition of potential threats through innate receptors, such as Toll-like receptors (TLRs) on the cell membrane and NOD-like proteins in the cytosol [19]. These receptors detect structural components common to bacteria or viruses, triggering signals that activate the expression of genes responsible for the synthesis of proinflammatory proteins, such as cytokines and inflammatory enzymes [20]. As a result, epithelial cells emit signals that can attract and activate leukocytes and increase blood flow and capillary permeability, among other responses. In addition, enterocytes can function as antigen-presenting cells, suggesting that their function goes beyond innate defence and participates in acquired immune responses [21].

The mucosal immune system is composed of three distinct anatomical compartments: organised structures such as Peyer patches and lymphoid follicles, the lamina propria and the surface epithelium [21]. The organised structures are sites of induction, while the lamina propria and epithelium contain mature and effector cells. The organised structures of the intestinal system are lined by a specialised epithelium that includes M cells, which facilitate the transport of micro-organisms or antigenic structures from the intestinal lumen to the underlying lymphoid tissue. Initiation of adaptive immune responses occurs primarily in the follicular structures of the intestinal mucosa. Here, processed antigens are presented to naïve T cells, triggering the expansion of lymphocyte clones with increased affinity for the antigen. This clonal expansion gives rise to different phenotypes of helper lymphocytes (Th cells), such as Th1, Th2 or regulatory T cells (Th3, Tr1 or CD4-CD25 cells). Regulatory T cells play a crucial role in immunotolerance by secreting cytokines with anti-inflammatory properties (such as IL-10 and TGF-beta) in response to antigens that are considered commensal and not pathogenic. Under normal conditions, the intestinal mucosa has a low number of activated T cells of Th1 phenotype, while regulatory T cells predominate. This immunotolerant situation allows continuous exposure to a considerable antigenic load, such as from bacterial flora and food, without triggering inflammatory reactions that may damage intestinal tissue [22, 23].

Interaction with the gut microbiome appears to be a key factor in the maintenance of this state of active immunotolerance, mediated by regulatory T cells [23]. Abnormalities in the development of the immune system could be related to defects in the interaction between the microbiota and the immuno-competent compartments of the intestinal mucosa. The hygiene hypothesis suggests that the increased incidence of allergic diseases, inflammatory bowel disease and autoimmune disorders in Westernised societies could be attributed to a reduction in exposure to microorganisms during the first months of life, including food-borne and orofaecal-borne helminths, which exerts a significant homeostatic impact [24].

4.1.3 Composition of the Gut Microbiota

Until recently, understanding of the gut microbiota was based on bacterial cultures of faecal samples, showing a predominance of anaerobic over aerobic bacteria. However, this method was limited, as many bacteria were not cultured in the laboratory. This questioned the true diversity and composition of the microbiota [5, 6].

Over the last two decades, various molecular biological techniques have been introduced to identify and characterise non-culturable bacteria [6]. These new technologies are providing entirely new insights into the gut ecosystem. For example, using electrophoresis, it is possible to separate bacterial DNA into bands, each representing bacterial groups with similar DNA sequences. Studies have revealed that each individual exhibits a characteristic and stable banding pattern over time, largely influenced by its genotype [25]. However, the influence of the environment is also observed, as in the case of individuals hospitalised in the same institution, who tend to lose diversity, especially under antibiotic treatment [26].

Some techniques use the sequence diversity of a bacterial gene, 16S ribosomal RNA, which allows for phylogenetic and taxonomic studies. These studies have revealed that each individual harbours a large number of unique strains, not shared with other individuals and previously unknown. In addition, new bacterial genera have been discovered that had previously gone unnoticed due to their difficulty in being isolated in laboratory culture. Moreover, these techniques have revealed differences in the predominant species between the proximal and distal third of the colon, as well as between the mucosal and faecal communities [27].

4.2 Dysfunctions of the Intestinal Microbiota and Diseases Associated with the Digestive Tract

Dysbiosis is an alteration of the gut microbiota and the adverse response of the host to these changes.

Several processes are associated with changes in the composition or metabolic function of the enteric flora [2].

4.2.1 Inflammatory Bowel Disease

This is a group of chronic disorders of the digestive system distinguished by the presence of inflammation whose cause has not yet been fully elucidated. Within this group, the two most common conditions are chronic ulcerative colitis (CUC) located in the colon and rectum and Crohn's disease (CD) located anywhere in the gastrointestinal tract. There is also a third group known as indeterminate colitis, which encompasses clinical symptoms shared by both diseases and can sometimes, over time, be diagnosed as one or the other [28].

As mentioned, the interaction between the structures of the gut mucosal immune system and the gut microbiome appears to be a major factor in the formation of the state of active immunotolerance mediated by regulatory T cells [23, 29–31]. Some abnormalities in the development of the immune system could be attributed to defects or inappropriate instructions of the regulatory pathways. Both Crohn's disease and ulcerative colitis are characterised by defects in regulatory T cell activity [32].

In Crohn's disease and ulcerative colitis, there is an abnormal activation of the mucosal immune system against elements of the enteric microbiome. This abnormal response appears to be the main trigger for the inflammatory mechanisms leading to intestinal injury [33]. In patients, increased mucosal secretion of IgG antibodies against commensal bacteria and hyper-reactivity of mucosal T lymphocytes to common flora antigens are observed, suggesting loss of local tolerance mechanisms [34, 35]. Indeed, in patients with Crohn's disease, diverting faecal flow may induce remission of lesions, whereas reintroducing intestinal contents into excluded ileal segments may reactivate the disease [36]. In ulcerative colitis, treatment of the colonic lumen with broad-spectrum antibiotics rapidly reduces inflammatory activity [37]. Genetic susceptibility and defects in the gut microbiome may be determinants for the development of inflammatory disease [38].

The lamina propria of the intestine is the site where immune system cells initially detect bacterial antigens. They then migrate to distal lymphoid tissues to trigger the inflammatory response [39]. Receptors on epithelial cells, such as Toll-like receptors and NOD2 receptors, play a crucial role in initiating the immune response.

When activated, these receptors can trigger an intracellular cascade leading to the production of proinflammatory cytokines [40]. This process promotes the maturation of mucosal dendritic cells, which, after contact with the antigen, migrate to local lymphoid structures, such as Peyer's patches, and head to the mesenteric nodes to initiate or maintain T cell and B cell responses. Dendritic cells are responsible for initiating the immune response, regulating intestinal inflammation and promoting tolerance. It is postulated that mucosal dendritic cells play a crucial role in regulating the immune response to the gastrointestinal antigenic load, thus maintaining intestinal homeostasis and allowing balanced coexistence with the endogenous microflora [39]. In healthy individuals, commensal flora generally fail to cross the intestinal epithelial barrier. However, when some bacteria do cross this barrier, they are rapidly phagocytosed by mucosal macrophages, which prevents activation of the intestinal immune response. Furthermore, when pathogenic microorganisms cross the barrier, an active immune response is triggered [41].

Some studies have found that a high proportion of bacteria present in faecal samples from patients with inflammatory disease belong to phylogenetic groups that are uncommon in healthy individuals [42]. Other studies show that patients with inflammatory disease have less species diversity in both faecal samples and the mucosa-associated bacterial community than healthy individuals [43]. Deficiency of a common commensal organism, Faecalibacterium prausnitzii, has been reported to be associated with early recurrence of Crohn's disease after surgery [44]. Low commensal species diversity is associated with ecosystem instability, which increases susceptibility to changes in ecosystem composition due to environmental influences. This ecosystem instability could favour temporary imbalances or alterations related to the risk of inflammation [45].

Patients with ulcerative colitis and Crohn's disease have a poorly diversified microbiota, with a predominance of *Clostridium*, *Bacteroides* and *Bifidobacteria* (commensal microbiota) and a concomitant increase in pathogenic bacteria, such as *Escherichia coli*, rare in individuals without inflammatory bowel involvement. The proportion of harmful bacteria could represent 30–40% of the dominant bacteria [46].

Treatment of IBD aims to control inflammation, relieve symptoms and prevent complications. Medications, such as anti-inflammatory drugs and immunosuppressants, may be prescribed depending on the severity of the disease. In severe cases or cases that do not respond to medical treatment, surgery may be necessary [47].

4.2.2 Coeliac Disease

Coeliac disease (CD) is now considered to be an immunologically mediated systemic disorder caused by gluten ingestion in genetically susceptible individuals and characterised by the presence of a variable combination of gluten-dependent clinical manifestations, disease-specific antibodies, HLA DQ2 or DQ8 haplotypes and enteropathy [48]. Withdrawal of gluten from the diet is associated with disappearance of symptoms and specific antibodies and normalisation of the intestinal mucosa in the vast majority of patients [49].

In coeliac patients, the immune response to gliadin fractions results in an inflammatory reaction, mainly in the upper small intestine, characterised by infiltration of the lamina propria and epithelium with inflammatory cells and villous atrophy. This response is mediated by innate and adaptive immunity. The adaptive response is mediated by CD4+ T cells in the lamina propria that recognise gliadin peptides, which bind to HLA class II molecules (DQ2 or DQ8) that are expressed on antigen presenting cells; the T cells subsequently produce pro-inflammatory cytokines, in particular interferon. The enzyme tissue transglutaminase deamidates gliadin peptides in the gut, increasing their immunogenicity [50].

Alterations in the gut microbiota of coeliac patients can increase the permeability of the intestine and trigger intense immune responses. This is due to changes in the gut lining, the mucus layer and the production of antimicrobial peptides. Toll-like receptors (TLRs) also play a key role in the immune response, while the gut microbiota may increase the production of inflammatory cytokines, contributing to the inflammatory profile of coeliac disease [51].

In addition to immunological and genetic factors, environmental factors, such as childhood nutrition and gut microbiota, are also suspected to play a role in the aetiopathogenesis of CD.

Studies in coeliac patients have shown that a strict gluten-free diet favours the reduction of beneficial bacterial colonies, especially *Bifidobacterium* and *Lactobacillus*, compared to gram-negative bacteria (*Bacteroides* and *E. coli*) [49]. This alteration of the microbiota due to gluten exclusion may be due to the elimination of important sources of carbohydrates, the main source of energy for the commensal microbiota. Dietary management of these patients does not support intestinal homeostasis; however, the suppressive immune response of the microbiota may be beneficial for CD patients [51].

4.2.3 Acute Diarrhoeal Diseases

Acute diarrhoea is a common gastrointestinal disorder characterised by loose or watery bowel movements and may be accompanied by other symptoms such as abdominal pain, fever, nausea and vomiting. It is defined as acute because it usually lasts less than 2 weeks and, in most cases, resolves on its own.

They are due to pathogens that proliferate and have invasive characteristics or produce toxins. Antibiotic-associated diarrhoea is due to an imbalance in the composition of the intestinal flora with the proliferation of pathogenic species, such as some toxin-producing strains of *Clostridium difficile* that cause pseudomembranous colitis.

In the treatment of patients with GEA, the priority is to rehydrate with oral solutions and reintroduce feeding rapidly. Rehydration with oral solutions helps to compensate for the loss of fluids and electrolytes caused by the disease. The use of probiotics is justified by their ability to change the composition of the gut microbiota, which prevents the growth of harmful bacteria that cause GEA [52].

4.2.4 *Helicobacter Pylori* Infection

More than 50% of the world's population is infected with *Helicobacter pylori*. Although the bacterial burden in the stomach is low, the *Helicobacter* species has received special attention due to its association with several gastric diseases. *H. pylori*, a gram-negative spirochaetal bacterium, is one of the most common causes of bacterial infection in humans, which can lead to gastritis, gastric and duodenal ulcer, stomach cancer and adenocarcinoma mucosal lymphoid tissue lymphoma, such as MALT-type lymphoma7 [53].

4.2.5 Obesity

Obesity results from increased consumption of foods high in energy, sugars and saturated fats; however, it appears that simply increasing calorie intake alone does not fully explain the current obesity epidemic. LG mice do not gain weight when exposed to high-fat and high-carbohydrate diets, suggesting that diet is not sufficient to induce obesity.

An "obese-type" human microbiota has been described, associated with excess weight and metabolic syndrome, with an increased *Firmicutes/Bacteroidetes* ratio [54]. *Bifidobacteria* and *Bacteroides* spp. appear to be protective against the development of obesity [55].

The ability to ferment dietary carbohydrates varies widely among microorganisms, and evidence points to a higher efficiency of the gut microbiota of overweight individuals to degrade non-digestible carbohydrates from vegetables. They showed that genetically obese (ob/ob) mice have 50% fewer *Bacteroidetes* and more *Firmicutes* than their lean siblings. They found that the microbiota of obese mice released more calories during digestion than those of lean mice. The obesity-generating phenotype may be transmissible [56].

These findings have led to the hypothesis that the microbiota of obese individuals may be more efficient in energy extraction than the microbiota of lean individuals. Some of the multiple metabolic mechanisms linking the microbiota to obesity and its related disorders, such as diabetes and fatty liver, include the following:

- Bacterial fermentation of dietary polysaccharides, which cannot be digested by the host, with consequent production of monosaccharides and SCFA. SCFA are substrates of colonocytes and precursors of cholesterol and fatty acids, substrates of gluconeogenesis in the liver, all of which optimise the utilisation of dietary energy.

- SCFA bind to specific receptors on intestinal endocrine cells (GRP43 and GRP41) that increase peptide YY, which slows intestinal transit, increase nutrient absorption and increase levels of leptin, an orexigenic hormone.
- Microbial regulation of some host genes that promote lipid deposition in adipocytes [57].
- Decreased intestinal expression of fasting-induced adipose factor (FIAF), also known as angiopoietin-like factor type iv, which is a circulating inhibitor of lipoprotein lipase that promotes fatty acid uptake and adipose tissue expansion. FIAF also induces peroxisome proliferator-activated receptor gamma coactivator 1, which regulates the expression of enzymes responsible for fatty acid oxidation [58]. Indeed, LG mice lacking the two alleles of FIAF have the same amount of body fat as conventional mice [57], so it is thought that FIAF may be a mediator of microbial regulation of peripheral fat stores [59].
- Obese mice have an increase in methanogenic archaea, which is associated with a lower partial pressure of hydrogen, which optimises the rate of bacterial fermentation [60].
- The microbiota increases inflammation-induced vascularisation and mucosal blood flow, which increases nutrient absorption [61].
- The gut microbiota is capable of promoting a state of low-grade systemic inflammation, insulin resistance and increased cardiovascular risk through mechanisms that include exposure to bacterial products, in particular LPS derived from gram-negative bacteria. This has been termed metabolic endotoxaemia [62]. They recently demonstrated an association between postprandial triglyceride levels and elevated bacterial endotoxins following a high-fat diet [63]. Changes in gut microbiota, increased intestinal permeability and endotoxaemia possibly play a role in the development of a chronic low-grade inflammatory state in the host that contributes to the development of obesity and chronic metabolic diseases, such as non-alcoholic fatty liver disease (NAFLD) [64].

4.2.6 Necrotising Enterocolitis

Necrotising enterocolitis (NEC) is the most common gastrointestinal emergency in newborns. It is a major clinical problem in newborns, affecting up to 10% of infants with a birth weight of less than 1500 g, especially those with very low birth weight (<1000 g) and those with a gestational age of less than 28 weeks [65]. The mortality rate is as high as 20–30% of victims. Morbidity is also high, especially neurodevelopmental changes in very-low-birth-weight infants [65, 66]. Despite advances in neonatal intensive care, NEC remains a potentially very severe disease in preterm infants without significant changes in the "status" of long-term mortality and morbidity [66].

Little is known about its pathogenesis. It has been associated with the presence of pathogenic bacteria, early hypoxia and the use of artificial milk, especially in relation to alterations in intestinal colonization. According to a recently published research [48], indicate that newborns affected by NEC show significant differences in their intestinal microbiota compared to other infants. In this study of nine newborns with NEC and nine other controls, a lower proportion of these bacteria was observed in patients with NEC compared to controls in the week prior to diagnosis [67]. These authors point out that without sufficient proteobacterial colonisation during the first week of life, preterm infants may be unable to regulate adaptive immune responses to subsequent proteobacterial growth [67]. Thus, imperfections in resistance mechanisms that affect the quality and quantity of the microflora may be associated with this disease.

4.2.7 Irritable Bowel Syndrome

Symptoms such as flatulence and flatulence are common in patients with IBS.

Significant differences have been demonstrated in the microbiota of IBS patients compared to healthy controls. A twofold increase in the *Firmicutes*/*Bacteroidetes* ratio was observed in patients [68]. IBS patients have lower amounts of *Lactobacillus* and *Bifidobacterium* spp. [69] than healthy controls. The aforementioned bacteria bind to epithelial cells and inhibit the binding of pathogenic bacteria, do not produce gas during carbohydrate fermentation and inhibit *Clostridia* spp. [70]. Probiotics change intestinal fermentation and stabilise the intestinal microflora. Over the last decade, studies have shown a link between IBS and bacterial overgrowth in breath tests using oral doses of lactulose or glucose.

CH4 is one of the gases present in the human gut and is produced by anaerobic bacterial fermentation. CH4 can affect the speed of intestinal transit and reduce serotonin secretion and has been associated with irritable bowel syndrome, diverticulosis and colorectal cancer [71]. The most important CH4-producing microorganism is *Methanobrevibacter smithii*, belonging to the *Archaea* domain [72]. CH4-producing adults have been shown to have longer intestinal transit times [73]. A recent study assessed CH4 production in 629 patients with intestinal symptoms using a breath glucose test. Of the patients, 32.3% were CH4 producers. This gas production may be significantly related to chronic constipation and was higher in patients with constipation compared to healthy subjects and significantly higher than in patients with diarrhoea [74].

4.2.8 Non-alcoholic Steatohepatitis/Non-alcoholic Fatty Liver Disease

Backhed demonstrated that regular collection of LG mice from the cecum of normal mice increased fatty liver disease [57]. NASH and NAFLD are associated with bacterial overgrowth and increased intestinal permeability, but not all studies are consistent [59].

Some bacterial products, including phenol, ammonia and ethanol, are potentially hepatotoxic [75]. Increased ethanol production has been reported in obese patients [76]. The main bacterial product associated with NASH and NAFLD is thought to be LPS, an active component of bacterial wall endotoxin, which is released when bacteria die in the gut. LPS undergoes capillary translocation and is absorbed along with dietary lipids through a TLR-4-dependent mechanism [77]. LPS absorption in turn activates the production of TNF-, IL-1 and IL-6. TLR-4-activated signalling promotes insulin resistance, hepatic steatosis, inflammation and fibrosis [75].

Chronic infusion of low-dose LPS in rats induces obesity and increased body fat percentage, insulin resistance, macrophage infiltration of adipose tissue and hepatic steatosis [78]. Human studies have shown that endotoxinemia is a risk factor for NAFLD. Two studies in patients diagnosed by biopsy showed a higher prevalence of endotoxinemia compared to healthy individuals [79, 80].

References

1. Palm NW, de Zoete MR, Flavell RA. Immune-microbiota interactions in health and disease. Clin Immunol. 2015;159(2):122–7.
2. Guarner F, Malagelada JR. Gut flora in health and disease. Lancet. 2003;361:512–9.
3. Eckburg PB, Bik EM, Bernstein CN, Purdom E, Dethlefsen L, Sargent M, Gill SR, Nelson KE, Relman DA. Diversity of the human intestinal microbial flora. Science. 2005;308(5728):1635–8.
4. Tannock GW. What immunologists should know about bacterial communities of the human bowel. Semin Immunol. 2006;19(2):94–105.
5. Suau A, Bonnet R, Sutren M, Godon JJ, Gibson G, Collins MD, Dore J. Direct rDNA community analysis reveals a myriad of novel bacterial lineages within the human gut. Appl Environ Microbiol. 1999;65(11):4799–807.
6. Zoetendal EG, Collier CT, Koike S, Mackie RI, Gaskins HR. Molecular ecological analysis of the gastrointestinal microbiota: a review. J Nutr. 2004;134(2):465–72.
7. Hooper LV, Wong MH, Thelin A, Hansson L, Falk PG, Gordon JI. Molecular analysis of commensal host-microbial relationships in the intestine. Science. 2001;291(5505):881–4.
8. Wostmann BS. The germfree animal in nutritional studies. Annu Rev Nutr. 1981;1:257–79.
9. Gill SR, Pop M, Deboy RT, Eckburg PB, Turnbaugh PJ, Samuel BS, Gordon JI, Relman DA, Fraser-Liggett CM, Nelson KE. Metagenomic analysis of the human distal gut microbiome. Science. 2006;312(5778):1355–9.
10. Hooper LV, Midtvedt T, Gordon JI. How host-microbial interactions shape the nutrient environment of the mammalian intestine. Annu Rev Nutr. 2002;22:283–307.
11. MacFarlane GT, Cummings JH, Allison C. Protein degradation by human intestinal bacteria. J Gen Microbiol. 1986;132(6):1647–56.
12. Smith EA, MacFarlane GT. Enumeration of human colonic bacteria producing phenolic and indolic compounds: effects of pH, carbohydrate availability and retention time on dissimilatory aromatic amino acid metabolism. J Appl Bacteriol. 1996;81(3):288–302.
13. Brook I. Bacterial interference. Crit Rev Microbiol. 1999;25(3):155–72.
14. Lievin V, Peiffer I, Hudault S, Rochat F, Brassart D, Neeser JR, Servin AL. Bifidobacterium strains from resident infant human gastrointestinal microflora exert antimicrobial activity. Gut. 2000;47(5):646–52.
15. Falk PG, Hooper LV, Midtvedt T, Gordon JI. Creating and maintaining the gastrointestinal ecosystem: what we know and need to know from gnotobiology. Microbiol Mol Biol Rev. 1998;62(4):1157–70.
16. Yamanaka T, Helgeland L, Farstad IN, Fukushima H, Midtvedt T, Brandtzaeg P. Microbial colonization drives lymphocyte accumulation and differentiation in the follicle-associated epithelium of Peyer's patches. J Immunol. 2003;170(2):816–22.

17. Helgeland L, Dissen E, Dai KZ, Midtvedt T, Brandtzaeg P, Vaage JT. Microbial colonization induces oligoclonal expansions of intraepithelial CD8 T cells in the gut. Eur J Immunol. 2004;34(12):3389–400.
18. Fagarasan S, Muramatsu M, Suzuki K, Nagaoka H, Hiai H, Honjo T. Critical roles of activation-induced cytidine deaminase in the homeostasis of gut flora. Science. 2002;298(5597):1424–7.
19. Aderem A, Ulevitch RJ. Toll-like receptors in the induction of the innate immune response. Nature. 2000;406(6797):782–7.
20. Elewaut D, DiDonato JA, Kim JM, y cols. NF-kappa B is a central regulator of the intestinal epithelial cell innate immune response induced by infection with enteroinvasive bacteria. J Immunol. 1999;163(3):1457–66.
21. Brandtzaeg PE. Current understanding of gastrointestinal immunoregulation and its relation to food allergy. Ann N Y Acad Sci. 2002;964:13–45.
22. Cummings JH, Antoine JM, Azpiroz F, Bourdet-Sicard R, Brandtzaeg P, Calder PC, Gibson GR, Guarner F, Isolauri E, Pannemans D, Shortt C, Tuijtelaars S, Watzl B. PASSCLAIM —gut health and immunity. Eur J Nutr. 2004;43(Suppl 2):II118–73.
23. Guarner F, Bourdet-Sicard R, Brandtzaeg P, Gill HS, McGuirk P, Van Eden W, Versalovic J, Weinstock JV, Rook GA. Mechanisms of disease: the hygiene hypothesis revisited. Nat Clin Pract Gastroenterol Hepatol. 2006;3(5):275–84.
24. Rook GA, Brunet LR. Microbes, immunoregulation, and the gut. Gut. 2005;54:317–20.
25. Zoetendal E, Akkermans A, Akkermans-van Vliet W, Visser J, de Vos W. The host genotype affects the bacterial community in the human gastrointestinal tract. Microbial Ecol Health Dis. 2001;13(3):129–34.
26. Bartosch S, Fite A, Macfarlane GT, McMurdo ME. Characterization of bacterial communities in feces from healthy elderly volunteers and hospitalized elderly patients by using real-time PCR and effects of antibiotic treatment on the fecal microbiota. Appl Environ Microbiol. 2004;70(6):3575–81.
27. Zoetendal EG, von Wright A, Vilpponen-Salmela T, Ben-Amor K, Akkermans ADL, de Vos WM. Mucosa-associated bacteria in the human gastrointestinal tract are uniformly distributed along the colon and differ from the community recovered from feces. Appl Environ Microbiol. 2002;68(7):3401–7.
28. Bentley D, Lifschitz C, Lawson M. Inflammatory bowel disease. In: Pediatric gastroenterology and clinical nutrition. London: Remedica; 2002.
29. Garrett WS, Gordon JI, Glimcher LH. Homeostasis and inflammation in the intestine. Cell. 2010;140(6):859–70.
30. Zak DE, Aderem A. Systems biology of innate immunity. Immunol Rev. 2009;227(1):264–82.
31. Björkstén B. Disease outcomes as a consequence of environmental influences on the development of the immune system. Curr Opin Allergy Clin Immunol. 2009;9(3):185–9.
32. Arif S, Tree TI, Astill TP, Tremble JM, Bishop AJ, Dayan CM, et al. Autoreactive T cell responses show proinflammatory polarization in diabetes but a regulatory phenotype in health. J Clin Invest. 2004;113(3):451–63.
33. Shanahan F. Inflammatory bowel disease: immunodiagnostics, immunotherapeutics, and ecotherapeutics. Gastroenterology. 2001;120(3):622–35.
34. Macpherson A, Khoo UY, Forgacs I, Philpott-Howard J, Bjarnason I. Mucosal antibodies in inflammatory bowel disease are directed against intestinal bacteria. Gut. 1996;38(3):365–75.
35. Pirzer U, Schönhaar A, Fleischer B, Hermann E, Meyer zum Büschenfelde KH. Reactivity of infiltrating T lymphocytes with microbial antigens in Crohn's disease. Lancet. 1991;338(8777):1238–9.
36. D'Haens GR, Geboes K, Peeters M, Baert F, Penninckx F, Rutgeerts P. Early lesions of recurrent Crohn's disease caused by infusion of intestinal contents in excluded ileum. Gastroenterology. 1998;114(2):262–7.
37. Casellas F, Borruel N, Papo M, Guarner F, Antolín M, Videla S, et al. Antiinflammatory effects of enterically coated amoxicillin-clavulanic acid in active ulcerative colitis. Inflammatory Bowel Dis. 1998;4(1):1–5.

38. Vermeire S. Review article: genetic susceptibility and application of genetic testing in clinical management of inflammatory bowel disease. Aliment Pharmacol Ther. 2006;24(Suppl 3):2–10.
39. Niess JH. Role of mucosal dendritic cells in inflammatory bowel disease. World Gastroenterol. 2008;14(33):5138–48.
40. Sansonetti PJ. War and peace at mucosal surfaces. Nat Rev Immunol. 2004;4(12):953–64.
41. Macpherson AJ, Gatto D, Sainsbury E, Harriman GR, Hengartner H, Zinkernagel RM. A primitive T cell-independent mechanism of intestinal mucosal IgA responses to commensal bacteria. Science. 2000;288(5474):2222–6.
42. Sokol H, Seksik P, Rigottier-Gois L, Lay C, Lepage P, Podglajen I, et al. Specificities of the fecal microbiota in inflammatory bowel disease. Inflamm Bowel Dis. 2006;12(2):106–11.
43. Frank DN, St Amand AL, Feldman RA, Boedeker EC, Harpaz N, Pace NR. Molecular—phylogenetic characterization of microbial community imbalances in human inflammatory bowel diseases. Proc Natl Acad Sci USA. 2007;104(34):13780–5.
44. Sokol H, Pigneur B, Watterlot L, Lakhdari O, BermúdezHumarán LG, Gratadoux JJ, et al. Faecalibacterium prausnitzii is an anti-inflammatory commensal bacterium identified by gut microbiota analysis of Crohn disease patients. Proc Natl Acad Sci USA. 2008;105(43):16731–6.
45. Martínez C, Antolín M, Santos J, Torrejón A, Casellas F, Borruel N, et al. Unstable composition of the fecal microbiota in ulcerative colitis during clinical remission. Am J Gastroenterol. 2008;103(3):643–8.
46. Danese S. Intestinal microbiota in inflammatory bowel disease: friend of foe. World J Gastroenterol. 2011;17(5):557–66.
47. Rowe FA, Walker JH, Karp LC, Vasiliauskas EA, Plevy SE, Targan SR. Factors predictive of response to cyclosporin treatment for severe steroid-resistant ulcerative colitis. Am J Gastroenterol. 2000;95(8):2000–8.
48. Husby S, Koletzko S, Korponay-Szabó IR, Mearin ML, Phillips A, Shamir R, et al. ESPGHAN working group on coeliac disease diagnosis; ESPGHAN gastroenterology committee. European Society for Pediatric Gastroenterology, hepatology, and nutrition guidelines for the diagnosis of coeliac disease. J Pediatr Gastroenterol Nutr. 2014;54(1):136–60.
49. Nadal I, Donat E, Ribes-Koninckx C, Calabuig M, Sanz Y. Imbalance in the composition of the duodenal microbiota of children with coeliac disease. J Med Microbiol. 2007;56(Pt 12):1669–74.
50. Polanco I. Celiac disease. J Pediatr Gastroenterol Nutr. 2008;47(Suppl 1):S3–6.
51. Laparra M, Olivares M, Sanz Y, Microbiota intestnal y enfermedad celíaca. En Rodrigo L y Peña AS, editores. Enfermedad celíaca y sensibilidad al gluten no celíaca. Barcelona, España: OmniaScience; 2013.
52. Szajewska H, Mrukowicz J. Meta-analysis: non-pathogenic yeast saccharomyces boulardii in the prevention of antibiotic-associated diarrhoea. Aliment Pharmacol Ther. 2005;22(5):365–72.
53. Asano N, Iijima K, Koike T, Imatani A, Shimosegawa T. Helicobacter pylori-negative gastric mucosa-associated lymphoid tissue lymphomas: a review. World J Gastroenterol. 2015;21(26):8014–20.
54. Raoult D. Obesity pandemics and the modification of digestive bacterial flora. Eur J Clin Microbiol Infect Dis. 2008;27(8):631–4.
55. Ley RE, Turnbaugh PJ, Klein S, et al. Microbial ecology: human gut microbes associated with obesity. Nature. 2006;444(7122):1022–3.
56. Turnbaugh PJ, Ley RE, Mahowald MA, et al. An obesity associated gut microbiome with increased capacity for energy harvest. Nature. 2006;444(7122):1027–31.
57. Backhed F, Ding H, Wang T, et al. The gut microbiota as an environmental factor that regulates fat storage. Proc Natl Acad Sci USA. 2004;101(44):15718–23.
58. Backhed F, Manchester JK, Semenkovich CF, et al. Mechanisms underlying the resistance to diet-induced obesity in germ-free mice. Proc Natl Acad Sci USA. 2007;104(3):979–84.
59. Machado MV, Cortez-Pinto H. Gut microbiota and nonalcoholic fatty liver disease. Ann Hepatol. 2012;11(4):440–9.

60. Ley RE, Backhed F, Turnbaugh P, et al. Obesity alters gut microbial ecology. Proc Natl Acad Sci USA. 2005;102(31):11070–5.
61. Ding S, Chi MM, Scull BP, et al. High-fat diet: bacteria interactions promote intestinal inflammation which precedes and correlates with obesity and insulin resistance in mouse. PLoS One. 2010;5(8):e12191.
62. Creely SJ, McTernan PG, Kusminski CM, et al. Lipopolysaccharide activates an innate immune system response in human adipose tissue in obesity and type 2 diabetes. Am J Physiol Endocrinol Metab. 2007;292(3):E740–7.
63. Clemente-Postigo M, Queipo-Ortuno MI, Murri M, et al. Endo- ˜ toxin increase after fat overload is related to postprandial hypertriglyceridemia in morbidly obese patients. J Lipid Res. 2012;53(5):973–8.
64. Fontana L, Eagton C, Trujillo ME, et al. Visceral fat adipokine secretion is associated with systemic inflammation in obese humans. Diabetes. 2007;56(4):1010–3.
65. Mihatsch WA, Braegger CP, Decsi T, Kolacek S, Lanzinger H, Mayer B, et al. Critical systematic review of the level of evidence for routine use of probiotics for reduction of mortality and prevention of necrotizing enterocolitis and sepsis in preterm infants. Clin Nutr. 2012;31(1):6–15.
66. Deshpande G, Rao S, Patole S, Bulsara M. Updated meta-analysis of probiotics for preventing necrotizing enterocolitis in preterm neonates. Pediatrics. 2010;125(5):921–30.
67. Mai V, Young CM, Ukhanova M, Wang X, Sun Y, Casella G, et al. Fecal microbiota in premature infants prior to necrotizing enterocolitis. PLoS One. 2011;6(6):e20647.
68. Alvarez-Llamas G, Szalowska E, de Vries MP. Characterization of the human visceral adipose tissue secretome. Mol Cell Proteomics. 2007;6(4):589–600.
69. Kassinen A, Krogius-Kurikka L, Makivuokko H, et al. The fecal microbiota of irritable bowel syndrome patients differs significantly from that of healthy subjects. Gastroenterology. 2007;133(1):24–33.
70. Spiller R. Review article: probiotics and prebiotics in irritable bowel syndrome. Aliment Pharmacol Ther. 2008;28(4):385–96.
71. Sahakian AB, Jee SR, Pimentel M. Methane and the gastrointestinal tract. Dig Dis Sci. 2010;55(8):2135–43.
72. Pochart P, Lemann F, Flourie B, et al. Pyxigraphic sampling to enumerate methanogens and anaerobes in the right colon of healthy humans. Gastroenterology. 1993;105(5):1281–5.
73. Stephen AM, Wiggins HS, Englyst HN, et al. The effect of age, sex and level of dietary fibre from wheat on large-bowel function in thirty healthy subjects. Br J Nutr. 1986;56(2):349–61.
74. Furnari M, Savarino E, Bruzzone L, et al. Reassessment of the role of methane production between irritable bowel syndrome and functional constipation. J Gastrointestin Liver Dis. 2012;21(2):157–63.
75. Abu-Shanab A, Quigley EM. The role of the gut microbiota in nonalcoholic fatty liver disease. Nat Rev Gastroenterol Hepatol. 2010;7(12):691–701.
76. Nair S, Cope K, Risby TH, Diehl AM. Obesity and female gender increase breath ethanol concentration: potential implications for the pathogenesis of nonalcoholic steatohepatitis. Am J Gastroenterol. 2001;96(4):1200–4.
77. Ghoshal S, Witta J, Zhong J, et al. Chylomicrons promote intestinal absorption of lipopolysaccharides. J Lipid Res. 2009;50(1):90–7.
78. Rivera CA, Adegboyega P, van Rooijen N, et al. Toll-like receptor-4 signaling and Kupffer cells play pivotal roles in the pathogenesis of non-alcoholic steatohepatitis. J Hepatol. 2007;47(4):571–9.
79. Thuy S, Ladurner R, Volynets V, et al. Nonalcoholic fatty liver disease in humans is associated with increased plasma endotoxin and plasminogen activator inhibitor 1 concentrations and with fructose intake. J Nutr. 2008;138(8):1452–5.
80. Harte AL, da Silva NF, Creely SJ, et al. Elevated endotoxin levels in non-alcoholic fatty liver disease. J Inflamma (Lond). 2010;7:15.

5 Microbiota and Diseases Associated with Rheumatic and Autoimmune Diseases

Alejandro Henar

5.1 Autoimmune and Rheumatic Diseases

Autoimmune diseases are a type of diseases that are characterized by the appearance of a special autoinflammatory process promoted by the generation of immunity against self-antigens. Usually, the immune system is in charge of generating an immunogenic response against potential risks to the organism such as bacteria or viruses that consist of detecting, attacking, and exterminating these risks. Knowing this, the immune system generates a tolerogenic response (a response in which the immune system "ignores" that antigen) against self-antigens thanks to various processes that inhibit or reduce the formation of so-called autoreactive T lymphocytes such as negative selection in the thymus, transformation of these autoreactive T lymphocytes into natural regulatory T lymphocytes (natural T REGs) in the thymus, or inducible regulatory T lymphocytes (inducible T REGs) in lymph nodes or mucosa-associated lymphoid tissues (MALT). B cells also undergo tolerance processes that mainly occur in the thymus. However, in autoimmune diseases, this regulation of autoimmunity is impaired, losing the tolerogenic response and leading to an autoimmune response. This response is produced mainly by an excess in autoreactive T and B lymphocytes that promote inflammation and generate antibodies (autoantibodies) against these own antigens, respectively.

Initiation of autoimmune response is often preceded by genetic susceptibilities (can also be non-genetic) to these diseases that, most commonly, cause an impaired thymic tolerance induction or an imbalance on pro- and anti-inflammatory signals. Already having this susceptibility, different initiating processes of autoimmunity can occur. Mainly they are processes that produce a modification of the processing mechanisms of self-antigens, modifications of self-antigens themselves, or formation of new self-antigens. Another of the most notable mechanisms that may induce

A. Henar (✉)
Department of Biomedicine, Universidad Alfonso X El Sabio, Madrid, Spain
e-mail: ahenaizq@myuax.com

J. Ruiz-Tovar (ed.), *Dysbiosis*, https://doi.org/10.1007/978-3-031-65650-7_5

an autoimmune response is antigen mimicry, which consists of the appearance of autoimmunity due to a cross-reaction with an infectious antigen; a prime example of this mechanism is Sjogren's syndrome, which is associated with Epstein-Barr virus infections.

On the other hand, rheumatic diseases are characterized by their involvement in the musculoskeletal system (joints, muscles, and connective tissues). Furthermore, some of these diseases can be classified within autoimmune diseases such as systemic lupus erythematosus (SLE) or antiphospholipid syndrome (APS), while others fall into the category of autoinflammatory diseases (without an autoimmune component) such as monogenic systemic autoinflammatory diseases (SAIDs). The main difference between autoimmune and autoinflammatory processes is the main agents of damage, while the principal cause of inflammation and damage in autoimmune diseases is the erroneous activation and self-targeting of the adaptive immune system; the damage in autoinflammatory diseases is done by the innate immune system due to abnormalities in regulatory mechanisms of the immune system, and little to no autoantibodies are generated in these diseases [1, 2].

However, not all rheumatic diseases can be classified as pure autoimmune or autoinflammatory diseases; some of them display a mixed pattern between them.

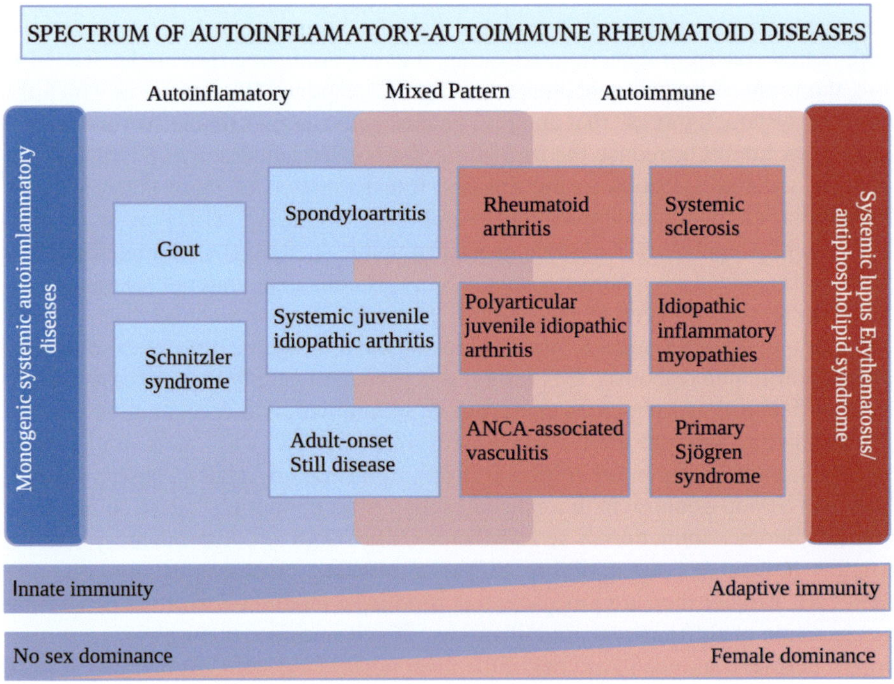

We can also observe that, as almost all other autoimmune diseases, more autoimmune-related rheumatic diseases tend to have a higher female dominance.

5.2 Role of Microbiota in Immunity Regulation

5.2.1 Microbiota and the Development of Gut-Associated Lymphoid Tissue (GALT)

One of the main connections between gut microbiota and the immune system is the GALT (gut-associated lymphoid tissue) which consist of several lymphatic structures that are present throughout the lower part of the digestive system. These structures include Peyer's patches, crypt patches, isolated lymphoid follicles (ILFs), appendix, and mesenteric lymph nodes (mLNs). Also related to immunity in the gut are M cells (which transfer antigens from the lumen of the intestine to the intratissue space), phagocytes (dendritic cells and macrophages), T lymphocytes, T REGs, B lymphocytes, and innate lymphoid cells (ILCs).

Moreover, development of GALT is highly mediated by lymphoid tissue inducer cells (LTi), a type of ILCs that, at the same time, need to interact with the gut commensal microorganisms to be able to do their function. This interaction is mediated mainly by Toll-like receptors (TLR), specifically TLR2; these proteins are the main type of pattern recognition receptors (PRR) and are responsible for detecting pathogen-associated molecular patterns (PAMP) found in foreign organisms. In the context of developing GALT, the recognition of commensal PAMPs promotes the activation of TLR pathways that promote the correct development of the lymphoid tissue and the generation of controlled immune tolerance against them mainly through specific molecules such as TLR2, nucleotide-binding oligomerization domain 1/2 (NOD 1/2), or TIR domain-containing adaptor protein inducing interferon (IFN)-β (TRIF). This is shown in several studies in which GALT development in mice without microbiota was studied. On top of this, studies have shown that commensal microorganism metabolites, mainly short-chain fatty acids (SCFAs), are also involved in GALT development through epigenetic mechanisms. Some studies have also shown that composition of gut microbiota alters molecule secretion of GALT which could translate in a higher or lower risk of generating autoimmune diseases [1–3].

5.2.2 Role of Conventional Natural Killer (cNK) Cells

One of the cells that may be more related to autoimmune diseases are conventional natural killer (cNK) cells; cNK cells are the only type of ILCs that have cytotoxic capabilities. One of the key features of these cells is their ability to differentiate between self and non-self; the process of how this cells obtain this ability is called education, and it is a major controversy field. The main theory is the "missing-self" theory that cNK cells recognize exogenous cells by detecting decreased expression of major histocompatibility complex (MHC) class I, but this can only partially explain the mechanism. In relation to this, different studies have shown that the absence of microbiota in mice results in cNK cells with a lower cytotoxic capacity; this leads to thinking that the molecules released by the microbiota to which these cells are exposed are involved in their development and possibly their education. Furthermore, it is reported that abnormal cNK cell phenotypes are common in several autoimmune diseases such as SLE or RA [1, 2, 4].

5.2.3 Role of Innate Lymphoid Cells (ILC)

Other cell types that could possibly be involved are ILC1, ILC2, and ILC3 cells, which function similarly to T helper cells, though, contrary to cNK cells, their development is independent of gut microbiota. The commensal microorganisms in the gut play a crucial role in priming specially ILC3s, enhancing their normal activities like cytokine secretion and antigen presentation. The absence or abnormality of the gut microbiota may disrupt the functioning of ILC3, potentially leading to overproliferation of pathogens or a breakdown in immune tolerance. This, in turn, could contribute to the development of autoimmune diseases, a connection that awaits confirmation through further research [1].

5.2.4 Role of Phagocytes (Macrophages and Dendritic Cells)

Phagocytes are also related to gut microbiota, in general, as already mentioned; short-chain fatty acids (SCFAs), produced by the gut microbiota, play a crucial role as a key regulator in the epigenetics of both local and distant immune systems. Existing knowledge suggests that signals derived from these microbiota-produced SCFAs are especially vital for maintaining the balance of phagocytes and restraining inflammatory responses through diverse mechanisms. The absence of SCFAs may increase the susceptibility to infection or inflammation-related diseases. On top of this, antigen-presenting cells such as dendritic cells play a pivotal role in connecting local immune responses to the microbiota and systemic autoimmunity. One significant mechanism involves antigens from altered microbiota, resembling self-tissue, presented by antigen-presenting cells, as strongly indicated by some metagenomics analysis. Furthermore, the gut microbiota might potentially induce distinct local immune responses of antigen-presenting cells, ultimately leading to altered adaptive immunity [1, 2].

5.2.5 Intestinal Permeability

An intricate relationship between intestinal microbiota, the immune system, and gut permeability has been identified, although not fully elucidated. The modulation of gut permeability is governed by the gut barrier, which includes the gut microbiota, mucus, enterocytes, tight junction (TJ) proteins, and innate and adaptive immune cells forming the gut-associated lymphoid tissue. The disassembly of TJ and the compromise of the intestinal barrier's integrity can result in increased intestinal permeability, allowing the passage of microbial antigens, products, or microorganisms themselves. TJ proteins, such as claudin-2, occludin, cingulin, and zonula occludens (ZO) proteins, regulate the TJ of the gut barrier. Moreover, there is evidence that intestinal permeability is influenced by elevated levels of zonulin, whose production is affected by bacterial colonization. Zonulin is known to reversibly regulate intestinal permeability by modulating TJ [5, 6].

Alterations in intestinal permeability can lead to leaky gut syndrome (LGS), which refers to an increased intestinal permeability and has been associated with the generation of an autoimmune response and a variety of autoimmune diseases. The main problems that arise from an increased intestinal permeability are an increased antigen exposure that can trigger an excessive immune reaction, especially in GALT and an alteration of the gut microbiota composition. Increase in TLR activation is very common in this situation, and in combination with all other factors, the risk of autoimmune reaction generation is substantially increased in these situations [5].

5.2.6 Microbiota Molecules' Role in Immune Modulation

There are several metabolites from the microbiota that exert regulatory effects on the immune system and inflammation. The most important of these metabolites are the aforementioned SCFAs, synthesized from inedible polysaccharides derived from proteins such as cellulose. The main SCFAs generated are acetate, propionate, and butyrate. For the most part, SCFAs bind to G protein-coupled receptors of the GPR family (GPR41, GPR43, and GPR 109A) and exert anti-inflammatory actions through epigenetic control of the homeostasis of T REGs.

Apart from metabolites, structural components such as polysaccharides also exert regulatory effects on immunity. The main example is the capsular polysaccharide A (PSA) of *Bacteroides fragilis* which, through its interaction with TLR2 of T REGs, regulates immunity in the intestine.

LPS (lipopolysaccharide) is also another molecule that is produced by gram-negative bacteria and that, in situations of gut dysbiosis where there is an overproduction, is capable of inducing a state of chronic inflammation [7].

5.3 Microbiota and Autoimmune Thyroid Diseases

Two main autoimmune thyroid diseases (AITD) exist, being Hashimoto's thyroiditis (HT) and Graves' disease (GD). In HT thyroid function decreases (hypothyroidism) due to the generation of autoantibodies that target thyroid peroxidase (TPO-Ab) or thyroglobulin (TG-Ab), main molecules involved in the thyroid hormone formation process. Contrary to this, patients with GD show a symptomatology of hyperthyroidism; this happens because autoantibodies generated in this disease target and activate thyroid receptors (TR-Ab) resulting in an increase in thyroid function. However, although these two diseases produce opposite symptoms, they share similar underlying immune-mediated mechanisms of disease and are related in many other areas such as genetic susceptibility [8, 9].

5.3.1 Microbiota Changes in Autoimmune Thyroid Diseases

In the last few years, several meta-analyses have been done to study the variation of microbiota in AITD patients. The results of these analyses show clear, significant changes between AITD patient microbiota and healthy patient microbiota [8, 9].

5.3.2 Changes in Alpha-Diversity

In a nutshell, Alpha-Diversity is a term that is based on richness (how many different species there are in an environment) and evenness (how evenly distributed they are). Generally speaking, higher diversity is commonly associated with healthier states. In relation to this, GD patients show a lower Alpha-Diversity than that of a healthy person, indicating association with several pathological conditions such as obesity, diabetes, inflammatory bowel diseases, polycystic ovary syndrome, and colorectal cancer. On the other hand, surprisingly, HT patients show an increase in their Alpha-Diversity; however, this connection may be linked to intestinal dysmotility, leading to prolonged gastrointestinal transit time and an increased risk of bacterial overgrowth in individuals with hypothyroidism. While greater microbiota diversity is generally associated with improved health outcomes, it can also have adverse effects, including heightened protein breakdown and reduced conversion of polyphenols, mucus secretion, and epithelial turnover [8, 9].

5.3.3 Changes in Relative Abundance

The two predominant phyla in the gut are *Firmicutes* and *Bacteroidetes*, and the ratio between these two (F/B) is an important metric that reveals the state of the gut microbiota, in addition to being an important marker of dysbiosis. What we can find in patients with GD is a decrease in the F/B ratio, mainly caused by a decrease in the number of *Bacteroidetes*. If we talk about genre, in GD patients, the most significant changes are, firstly, the decrease in *Bacteroidetes*, bacteria that ferment glucose and lactate, thus generating SCFAs that promote intestinal barrier stability; because of this, lack of these bacteria can produce leaky gut syndrome (LGS). On top of this, there is also an increase in the amount of *Prevotella*, species known for their activation of TLR2 and consequently for their role in mucosal inflammation. To a lesser extent, increases in the amount of *Actinobacteria* and *Collinsella* also occur. On the other hand, *Lactobacillus* and *Bifidobacterium*, genres that are associated with healthy microbiota, were underrepresented. It is important to note that HT patients do show similar variation in relative abundance but to a lesser extent compared with healthy individuals, and this may imply a lesser importance of gut microbiota in this disease [8, 9].

5.4 Microbiota and Type 1 Diabetes

Type 1 diabetes (T1D) is the second most common type of diabetes and, in contrast to type 2 diabetes, has an autoimmune origin. The autoimmune reaction is characterized by the development of reactive T cells and autoantibodies that target the Langerhans cells of the pancreatic islets, cells whose main function is the synthesis and secretion of insulin, an essential hormone in cellular metabolism, especially in carbohydrate anabolism. Type 1 diabetes has a very studied and very important genetic component, but in recent years it has also been shown that alterations in the gut microbiota, increases in intestinal permeability, and intestinal inflammation have a certain relationship with the disease. Another relationship between the microbiota of the gut and the intestine is its lymphatic connection, since both the duodenum and the pancreas are drained by the same lymph node system (among which are the pancreatic lymph node and the duodenal lymph node); alterations in homeostasis in the duodenum can produce alterations in the pancreas through the lymphatic system [5, 6, 10].

5.4.1 Gut Microbiota Dysbiosis in T1D

In type 1 diabetes (T1D), the observed changes in gut microbiota composition and a decrease in alpha-diversity, such as an increased *Firmicutes*/*Bacteroidetes* ratio, elevated *Bacteroides* and *Enterobacteriaceae* levels, and reductions in beneficial bacteria like *Faecalibacterium prausnitzii*, *Bifidobacterium* species, and *Akkermansia muciniphila* are of significance due to their potential implications for host health. *Faecalibacterium prausnitzii*, known for butyrate production, contributes to gut mucosal integrity and anti-inflammatory effects. *Bifidobacterium* species play a crucial role in maintaining gut health and have immunomodulatory properties. *Akkermansia muciniphila* is associated with mucosal barrier function. Alterations in these microbial components can impact metabolic functions, immune responses, and gut barrier integrity, potentially influencing the autoimmune processes underlying T1D [6, 10].

5.4.2 Gut Microbiota Dysbiosis Autoimmune Inducing Mechanisms

What seems to be the main mechanism that can drive the autoimmune reaction is the decrease in intestinal permeability. There is also the hypothesis that some commensal bacteria can induce a cross-reactivity process between the GAD (glutamic acid decarboxylase) of the commensal bacteria and human GAD (one of the main autoantigens in T1D) that ends up in the formation of GADAs (glutamic acid decarboxylase antibodies). Something similar can also occur with peptide sequences similar to that of insulin found in some gut bacteria such as various species of *Bacteroides* and *Clostridium*. Also, as mentioned before, to these mechanisms is added the decrease in species that produce SCFAs (mainly butyrate) [5, 6].

5.5 Microbiota in Autoimmune Liver Diseases

Primary biliary cholangitis (PBC) and autoimmune hepatitis (AIH) are the main two autoimmune liver diseases. Although they are grouped in the same category, their pathophysiologies are only similar in their autoimmune origin, and as many other autoimmune diseases, the initiation of these two pathologies is thought to occur when a specific environmental factor triggers an autoimmune reaction in genetically susceptible individuals; however, the underlying mechanisms of pathogenesis are not fully understood [11].

5.5.1 Microbiota in Autoimmune Hepatitis

Main changes in microbiota in AIH can be found both in gut and oral microbiota. *Veillonella dispar* is a bacteria species that is overrepresented in AIH patients in oral microbiota and stimulates secretion of proinflammatory cytokines such as IL-1β, IL-6, IL-8, and IL-12p70 that can be found in higher quantities than normal in saliva. On the other hand, *Lactobacillales* species, another inflammation-inducing bacteria, are overrepresented in gut microbiota of AIH patients and are positively correlated with *Veillonella* levels in saliva [11, 12].

5.5.2 Microbiota in Primary Biliary Cholangitis

A notable feature in individuals with PBC is decreased microbial diversity being a common observation. One specific trend involves an elevated abundance of bacteria within the *Proteobacteria* phylum, notably associated with inflammation. The expanded presence of *Proteobacteria* in the gut of PBC patients raises questions about its potential role in contributing to the inflammatory processes associated with the disease. Moreover, the alterations extend beyond phylum-level changes, impacting the production of key bacterial metabolites. The gut microbiota's role in bile acid metabolism, for instance, is of particular interest in the context of PBC, given the central role of bile ducts in the disease pathology [13].

5.6 Microbiota and Rheumatoid Arthritis (RA)

RA is a systemic autoimmune rheumatic disease that specially affects joints causing synovitis; it also has an autoinflammatory origin, meaning that the chronic inflammation is caused both by the innate and adaptive system. The main alterations can be found in excessive Th17 cell response, excessive macrophage response, and excessive activation of the inflammasome; this leads to an increase in IL17 (Th17), IL, TNF-α, IL6 (macrophages), IL1-β, and IL18 (inflammasome) all of which are pro-inflammatory cytokines and in addition to autoreactive Tc and B cell generation. These alterations are mainly observed in synovium and synovial fluid (joints) [1, 14].

5.6.1 Role of Microbiota

RA may be the disease in which microbiota has been most studied thanks to a lot of studies that support this idea. Knowing this, alterations in the composition of intestinal bacteria in individuals with preclinical and established RA suggest a vital role of the gut microbiota in immune dysfunction characteristic of RA, and various studies have shown that salivary, dental, and fecal microbiota diversity in patients with RA is significantly different to those without RA, and at the same time, this diversity alteration is also correlated with symptomatology and autoantibody production [15, 16].

The mechanisms in which microbiota can initiate an autoimmune response are triggered through dysbiosis. It has been seen that, at the beginning of RA, several species of bacteria increase, while others decrease. The main ones that increase are *Prevotella* and *Lactobacillus*, while those that decrease are mainly *Bacteroidetes* and *Bifidobacteria*. This change in diversity induces the local activation of both the innate system and self-reactive adaptive cells and, therefore, the generation of an autoimmune response that ends up migrating to the joints [16–18].

This demonstrates the important role of gut microbiota in the development of the disease. Specifically, the main molecules that may contribute to the pathophysiology of the disease are the activation of certain TLR-PAMP pairs. One possible important TLR in this area is TLR4. Activation of TLR4 gives rise to an increase in inflammation in the affected joints mediated by an increase in survival and consequently the number of Th17 cells, which produces an increase in IL17. This happens because the activation of TLR4 produces an increase in both IL1 and IL23, which promotes the survival of Th17 cells [1, 14].

The inflammasome may also be an important key component in RA and microbiota. Evidence suggests that, as already mentioned, proinflammatory cytokines induced by inflammasome activation are a major component of RA [19]. Furthermore, there is evidence of a relationship with certain polymorphisms of proteins related to the inflammasome such as NLRP3 and CARD8 and RA [1].

Another mechanism involved in the generation of autoimmunity is the possible loss of intestinal barrier function due to different types of bacteria. This can be seen in overrepresented and underrepresented species of commensal bacteria in RA patients; main examples are *Collinsella aerofaciens* (overrepresented) and *Faecalibacterium prausnitzii* (underrepresented) which promote intestinal barrier dysfunction and protect from intestinal barrier dysfunction, respectively [16, 20].

Regarding antigen mimicry, in more than 50% of patients with RA, autoreactive T and B cells can be found against the autoantigens *N*-acetylglucosamine-6-sulfatase and filamin A. These autoantigens have homologous sequences with protein epitopes of the species *Prevotella*, *Parabacteroides*, and *Butyricimonas*. Another possible candidate is the *Collinsella* species that has sequences homologous to the DRB1*0401 autoantigen [16].

5.6.2 Possible Diagnostic Uses of Gut Microbiota in RA

In the early diagnosis of rheumatoid arthritis (RA), studies suggest an increased presence of *Prevotella copri* and a decrease in *Bacteroidetes*, which are associated with early RA. Additionally, there was an observed increase in *Lactobacillus* in early RA patients. During the active, advanced phase of RA, the reduction of *Haemophilus* spp. correlated negatively with disease severity, while *Lactobacillus salivarius* increased in cases of very active RA. On top of this, higher levels of *Collinsella* and *Akkermansia* are present in active RA patients. These microbiota changes could serve as diagnostic markers, but further research is needed for confirmation [16, 18, 20].

5.7 Microbiota and Systemic Lupus Erythematosus (SLE)

Systemic lupus erythematosus (SLE) represents a multifaceted autoimmune disorder characterized by the production of autoantibodies and widespread inflammation that gives rise to a spectrum of symptoms affecting diverse organs and systems. Clinical manifestations include joint pain; distinctive skin rashes, particularly the butterfly-shaped rash; renal complications; and profound fatigue. The etiology of lupus remains intricate, involving a confluence of genetic predispositions, environmental triggers, and hormonal influences. Recent investigations have delved into the relationship between lupus and the microbiota, exploring potential connections between alterations in the microbial community and the onset or exacerbation of autoimmune conditions [5, 21].

5.7.1 Changes in SLE Patient's Microbiota

Just like what happens with the microbiota in the other autoimmune diseases that we have already talked about, the F/B index is altered; in this case, an increase in the index has been seen due to a decrease in the abundance of *Firmicutes*; this change suggests a negative correlation between the disease and the number of *firmicutes* and therefore also suggests a possible protective role of this phyla. In addition to this, the diversity and richness of the gut microbiota are decreased in patients with SLE compared to healthy people. It should also be noted that, specifically, the abundance of *Ruminococcus gnavus* in patients with SLE increases by fivefold, which is also correlated with an increase in anti-*Ruminococcus* antibodies in the patients' serum [5, 21].

5.8 Microbiota and Multiple Sclerosis

Multiple sclerosis is an autoimmune disease that affects the central nervous system. As in other autoimmune diseases, autoreactive cells are generated, in this case mainly Th1 and Th17 cells, which produce inflammation and tissue damage mainly through the release of several cytokines such as IFN-γ and IL17. The main consequence of this autoimmune reaction is demyelination and consequent neurodegeneration [5, 22].

5.8.1 Alterations in Gut Microbiota and Intestinal Permeability

In the interplay between the gut microbiota and multiple sclerosis (MS), emerging scientific investigations have unveiled specific alterations in microbial species that may contribute to the pathogenesis and progression of this autoimmune disorder.

Noteworthy among these microbial actors is *Prevotella*, whose reduced abundance in individuals with MS has been correlated with an attenuation of its immunomodulatory properties. *Prevotella*'s capacity to generate short-chain fatty acids suggests a potential role in shaping the immune response relevant to MS. The *Firmicutes* phylum, particularly the presence of *Faecalibacterium*, assumes a prominent role thanks to its generation of SCFAs, specifically for its butyrate production. Reduced levels of *Faecalibacterium* have been observed in the gut microbiota of individuals with MS, producing a deficit in butyrate-producing bacteria. *Akkermansia muciniphila* is an intriguing participant. While findings regarding its abundance in MS are not universally consistent, some studies posit an elevated presence in affected individuals. *Akkermansia*'s role in mucin degradation raises questions about its potential impact on gut barrier function. Perturbations in mucosal integrity, influenced by alterations in *Akkermansia* abundance, may play a role in fostering an environment conducive to inflammation and immune dysregulation, both hallmark features of MS.

Beyond these individual microbial actors, the broader theme of changes in microbial diversity and composition emerges as a focal point in the investigation of the MS-associated microbiota. Individuals with MS frequently exhibit a reduction in overall microbial diversity, indicative of a dysbiosis that extends beyond specific taxa. This microbial imbalance may contribute substantially to the complex and dynamic relationship between the gut microbiota and the pathophysiology of MS [5, 22].

5.9 Precision Medicine in Microbiota and Autoimmune Diseases

5.9.1 Microbiota Biomarkers

Ongoing research aims to identify specific microbiota biomarkers associated with autoimmune diseases. The presence or absence of certain bacterial strains, along with the overall diversity of the microbiome, is being studied for its role in predisposition or the onset of autoimmune diseases. Knowing this, the identification of reliable microbiome biomarkers holds promise for early diagnosis and personalized treatment strategies.

Integration of precision medicine in this topic is based on the development of different therapies such as tailored therapies; precision medicine strategies seek to tailor interventions based on an individual's unique microbiota profile, allowing for more targeted and effective treatments. For example, if a person with rheumatoid arthritis has a specific imbalance in their gut microbiota, a tailored therapy might involve prescribing a probiotic regimen designed to restore balance. Other therapeutic approaches may be based on integrating individual microbiota information into treatment plans and may involve personalized probiotic regimens, prebiotic supplementation, or even fecal microbiota transplantation (FMT) to address specific microbial imbalances. In the case of inflammatory bowel disease, a patient with identified microbiota imbalances may receive a personalized treatment plan that includes specific prebiotics to foster the growth of beneficial bacteria.

5.9.2 Impact on the Immune System

As already discussed, the microbiota plays a pivotal role in educating and regulating the immune system, particularly within the gut. Understanding a patient's unique microbiota educational profile could inform healthcare providers about potential immune system dysregulations, guiding them to develop more immune targeted treatment strategies.

In order to be able to modulate the immune response through the microbiota, new knowledge of specific microbiota-immune cell interactions should be acquired, and this could lead to the development of therapies that modulate immune responses in autoimmune diseases, such as lupus.

5.9.3 Microbiota Therapies in Autoimmune Diseases

- Probiotics: Studies explore the use of probiotics, beneficial microorganisms, to restore a balanced microbiota and potentially alleviate autoimmune symptoms. For instance, a patient with rheumatoid arthritis may be prescribed a specific probiotic strain known to have anti-inflammatory properties.

- Prebiotics: Substances promoting the growth of beneficial bacteria, known as prebiotics, are investigated for their role in shaping a healthier gut microbiome. Personalized prebiotic recommendations could be provided to individuals with autoimmune conditions to support the growth of beneficial microbes.
- Fecal microbiota transplantation (FMT): FMT is being researched as a more advanced approach to reset the gut microbiota, with potential applications in autoimmune disease management. If a patient with an autoimmune disease has a severely disrupted microbiota, FMT may be considered to restore a healthy microbial balance.

5.9.4 Mouse Models

Studies in mouse models have provided valuable insights into how manipulating the microbiota can affect susceptibility to autoimmune diseases. These insights may guide the development of targeted interventions in humans based on the observed effects in mouse models. Precision medicine approaches in mouse models involve tailoring interventions based on the specific genetic and microbiota profiles of individual mice. For instance, identifying distinct microbiota patterns associated with susceptibility or resistance to autoimmune conditions in genetically modified mice allows for precise interventions that mimic individualized responses.

Microbiota-genetics interactions can be studied as a part of precision medicine. Translating this knowledge to humans could lead to personalized interventions that consider an individual's unique genetic and microbial landscape, influencing susceptibility or resilience to autoimmune diseases. Similarly, targeted therapy studies as a form of precision medicine may allow for the development of personalized targeted therapies in patients. For example, if a specific microbiota manipulation proves effective in a genetically defined group of mice, a similar approach could be explored in a subset of patients with similar genetic and microbiota profiles, offering a more precise and tailored treatment strategy.

5.9.5 Microbiota and Treatment Response

Treatment personalization is the main objective of precision medicine. However, variability in microbiota composition is a major factor being explored that influences how individuals respond to conventional treatments for autoimmune diseases. Identifying an individual's microbiota profile can help predict their response to standard treatments, allowing for adjustments or alternative approaches if needed.

5.9.6 Challenges and Future Research

Standardization of microbiome analysis methods remains a challenge, and concerted efforts are required to establish robust and reproducible methods. A standardized approach is important to ensure the reliability of microbiome data used in precision medicine applications. Additionally, addressing individual differences in microbiota responses remains a major challenge, and further research into the factors that influence individual responses is required. This ongoing research will help refine precision medicine approaches tailored to changes in an individual's microbiome. Future research will aim to better understand the precise patterns of the microbiota and uncover the complex mechanisms that control the interaction between the microbiota and the immune system. This advanced understanding may pave the way for more targeted and effective precision medicine interventions for autoimmune diseases. This comprehensive review has highlighted the complex relationship between the microbiota and autoimmune diseases and demonstrates the promising potential of personalized interventions in the dynamic context of precision medicine [1, 5, 11, 16, 23].

References

1. Szekanecz Z, McInnes IB, Schett G, Szamosi S, Benkő S, Szűcs G. Autoinflammation and autoimmunity across rheumatic and musculoskeletal diseases. Nat Rev Rheumatol. 2021;17(10):585–95. https://pubmed.ncbi.nlm.nih.gov/34341562/
2. Shin JI, Lee KH, Joo YH, Lee JM, Jeon J, Jung HJ, et al. Inflammasomes and autoimmune and rheumatic diseases: a comprehensive review. J Autoimmun. 2019;103:102299. https://pubmed.ncbi.nlm.nih.gov/31326231/
3. Erkeller-Yuksel F, Lydyard P, Isenberg D. Lack of NK cells in lupus patients with renal involvement. Lupus. 1997;6:708–12. https://doi.org/10.1177/096120339700600905.
4. Stanisavljević S, Lukić J, Momčilović M, Miljković M, Jevtić B, Kojić M, et al. Gut-associated lymphoid tissue, gut microbes and susceptibility to experimental autoimmune encephalomyelitis. Benef Microbes. 2016;7:363–73. https://doi.org/10.3920/BM2015.0159.
5. Christovich A, Luo XM. Gut microbiota, leaky gut, and autoimmune diseases. Front Immunol. 2022;13:946248. https://www.frontiersin.org/articles/10.3389/fimmu.2022.946248/full
6. Del Chierico F, Rapini N, Deodati A, Matteoli MC, Cianfarani S, Putignani L. Pathophysiology of type 1 diabetes and gut microbiota role. Int J Mol Sci. 2022;23(23):14650. https://www.mdpi.com/1422-0067/23/23/14650
7. Shapiro H, Thaiss CA, Levy M, Elinav E. The cross talk between microbiota and the immune system: metabolites take center stage. Curr Opin Immunol. 2014;30:54–62. https://pubmed.ncbi.nlm.nih.gov/25064714/
8. Gong B, Wang C, Meng F, Wang H, Song B, Yang Y, et al. Association between gut microbiota and autoimmune thyroid disease: a systematic review and meta-analysis. Front Endocrinol (Lausanne). 2021;12:774362. https://www.frontiersin.org/articles/10.3389/fendo.2021.774362/full
9. Chen B, Jia X-m, Xu J-y, Zhao L-d, Ji J-y, Wu B-x, et al. Proinflammatory and autoimmunogenic gut microbiome in systemic lupus erythematosus. bioRxiv. 2019:621995. https://doi.org/10.1101/621995.
10. Vatanen T, Franzosa EA, Schwager R, Tripathi S, Arthur TD, Vehik K, Lernmark Å, Hagopian WA, Rewers MJ, She J-X, et al. The human gut microbiome in early-onset type 1 diabetes from the TEDDY study. Nature. 2018;562:589–94. https://doi.org/10.1038/s41586-018-0620-2.
11. Abe K, Fujita M, Hayashi M, Okai K, Takahashi A, Ohira H. Gut and oral microbiota in autoimmune liver disease. Fukushima J Med Sci. 2020;65(3):71–5. https://www.jstage.jst.go.jp/article/fms/65/3/65_2019-21/_article

12. Abe K, Takahashi A, Fujita M, Imaizumi H, Hayashi M, Okai K, et al. Dysbiosis of oral microbiota and its association with salivary immunological biomarkers in autoimmune liver disease. PLoS One. 2018;13(7):e0198757.
13. Tang R, Wei Y, Li Y, Chen W, Chen H, Wang Q, Yang F, Miao Q, Xiao X, Zhang H, Lian M, Jiang X, Zhang J, Cao Q, Fan Z, Wu M, Qiu D, Fang JY, Ansari A, Gershwin ME, Ma X. Gut microbial profile is altered in primary biliary cholangitis and partially restored after UDCA therapy. Gut. 2018;67:534–41.
14. Abdollahi-Roodsaz S, Joosten LAB, Koenders MI, Devesa I, Roelofs MF, Radstake TRDJ, et al. Stimulation of TLR2 and TLR4 differentially skews the balance of T cells in a mouse model of arthritis. J Clin Invest. 2008;118(1):205–16. http://content.the-jci.org/articles/view/32639
15. Sun Y, Chen Q, Lin P, Xu R, He D, Ji W, et al. Characteristics of gut microbiota in patients with rheumatoid arthritis in Shanghai, China. Front Cell Infect Microbiol. 2019;9:369. https://doi.org/10.3389/fcimb.2019.00369.
16. Zhao T, Wei Y, Zhu Y, Xie Z, Hai Q, Li Z, et al. Gut microbiota and rheumatoid arthritis: from pathogenesis to novel therapeutic opportunities. Front Immunol. 2022;13:1007165. https://www.frontiersin.org/articles/10.3389/fimmu.2022.1007165/full
17. Pianta A, Arvikar S, Strle K, Drouin EE, Wang Q, Costello CE, et al. Evidence of the immune relevance of Prevotella copri, a gut microbe, in patients with rheumatoid arthritis. Arthritis Rheumatol. 2017;69:964–75. https://doi.org/10.1002/art.40003.
18. Maeda Y, Kurakawa T, Umemoto E, Motooka D, Ito Y, Gotoh K, et al. Dysbiosis contributes to arthritis development via activation of autoreactive T cells in the intestine. Arthritis Rheumatol. 2016;68(11):2646–61. https://doi.org/10.1002/art.39783.
19. Martinon F, Burns K, Tschopp J. The inflammasome: a molecular platform triggering activation of inflammatory caspases and processing of proIL-β. Mol Cell. 2002;10:417–26. https://doi.org/10.1016/S1097-2765(02)00599-3.
20. Scher JU, Sczesnak A, Longman RS, Segata N, Ubeda C, Bielski C, et al. Expansion of intestinal Prevotella copri correlates with enhanced susceptibility to arthritis. elife. 2013;2:e01202. https://doi.org/10.7554/eLife.01202.
21. Pan Q, Guo F, Huang Y, Li A, Chen S, Chen J, et al. Gut microbiota dysbiosis in systemic lupus erythematosus: novel insights into mechanisms and promising therapeutic strategies. Front Immunol. 2021;12:799788. https://www.frontiersin.org/articles/10.3389/fimmu.2021.799788/full
22. Berer K, Mues M, Koutrolos M, AlRasbi Z, Boziki M, Johner C, et al. Commensal microbiota and myelin autoantigen cooperate to trigger autoimmune demyelination. Nature. 2011;479:28484. https://doi.org/10.1038/nature10554.
23. Yang W, Yu T, Cong Y. CD4+ T cell metabolism, gut microbiota, and autoimmune diseases: implication in precision medicine of autoimmune diseases. Precis Clin Med. 2022;5(3):bac018. https://academic.oup.com/pcm/article/doi/10.1093/pcmedi/pbac018/6632993

Microbiota and Diseases Associated with Metabolic Syndrome

6

Esther Lluch-Bataller

6.1 Introduction

6.1.1 Definition of Metabolic Syndrome

Metabolic syndrome (MS) is considered one of the most relevant complex diseases of the twenty-first century. Metabolic syndrome refers to a set of metabolic alterations framed within the context of **chronic inflammation** and **insulin resistance** (IR). MS is a group of conditions that collectively increase the risk of coronary heart disease, diabetes, stroke, and other serious health issues.

MS is a **multifactorial** disease related to various biochemical alterations stemming from oxidative stress, inflammation, and dysbiosis. This process is characterized by a disorder originating from chronic adiposity-based disease (CAD) and is defined by increased visceral adipose tissue, decreased high-density lipoprotein (HDL) concentrations, elevated triglyceride and low-density lipoprotein (LDL) concentrations, endothelial dysfunction with increased blood pressure, and chronic hyperglycemia.

The **etiology** of MS is often linked to central or visceral obesity as a determinant factor of insulin resistance. However, other factors such as genetics and environmental influences are also crucial for the development of this syndrome, with dietary habits being one of the main factors. High intake of simple carbohydrates and saturated fatty acids, coupled with low consumption of fruits and vegetables, is cited as contributing factors. Malnutrition and genetic factors play pivotal roles in the development of obesity, insulin resistance, and, consequently, metabolic syndrome.

Metabolic syndrome encompasses at least three of the following conditions (Fig. 6.1):

E. Lluch-Bataller (✉)
Department of Biomedicine, Universidad Alfonso X EL Sabio, Madrid, Spain
e-mail: esther.lluch.bataller@gmail.com

J. Ruiz-Tovar (ed.), *Dysbiosis*, https://doi.org/10.1007/978-3-031-65650-7_6

- **Abdominal obesity**: Excess abdominal fat is a significant risk factor for developing heart disease.
- **High blood pressure**: Prolonged high blood pressure can damage the heart and blood vessels, increasing the risk of atherosclerotic plaque buildup and thus the risk of heart disease or strokes.
- **High serum glucose levels**: This can damage blood vessels and increase the risk of developing diabetes.
- **High serum triglyceride levels**: Elevated triglyceride levels can raise LDL cholesterol levels, consequently increasing the risk of heart diseases.
- **Low HDL cholesterol**: Adequate blood cholesterol levels are crucial for heart health. HDL cholesterol works to remove LDL cholesterol from blood vessels, which could otherwise lead to plaque buildup in the blood vessels (Fig. 6.1).

Publications worldwide demonstrate the current importance of diagnosing and preventing metabolic syndrome. Various analyses concluded that patients with MS had twice the risk of mortality from cardiovascular causes and 1.5 times the risk from all etiologies. In general terms, it can be affirmed that one in every three or four individuals over 20 years old meets the criteria for an MS diagnosis.

The prevalence increases with age, is more common in women, and has significantly risen in the last decade, with a higher number of cases in the young population. This epidemic trend can be explained by various factors such as race,

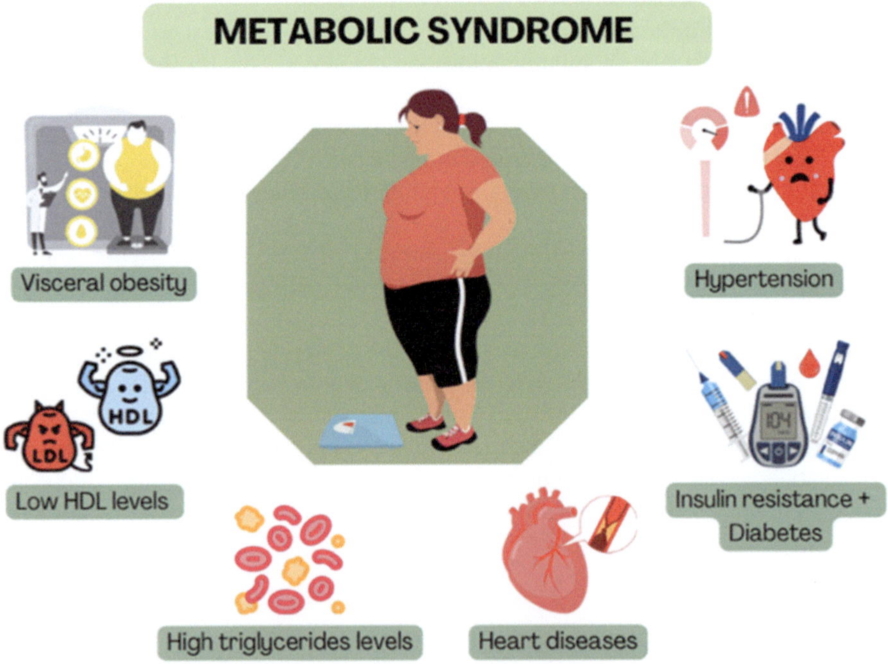

Fig. 6.1 Representation of the various conditions of metabolic syndrome

malnutrition, population aging, changes in lifestyle, urbanization processes, and sedentary behavior. These factors culminate in a cluster of **metabolic abnormalities**, such as type 2 diabetes mellitus, altered fasting glucose, high blood pressure, hyperlipidemia, obesity, and microalbuminuria (Fig. 6.2).

The **pathophysiology** of metabolic syndrome encompasses alterations in glucolipid metabolism, proinflammatory, and prothrombotic states. The link between these alterations is attributed to insulin resistance, favored by increased free fatty acids, often associated with overweight. This condition leads to disruptions in cellular glucose utilization and deregulation of hepatic glucose production.

Lipid metabolism also shows consequences of insulin resistance, resulting in characteristic alterations of MS: **hypertriglyceridemia** and **low HDL cholesterol**.

Moreover, **hypertension** is related to different mechanisms as a consequence of alterations in the insulin pathway and the regulation of the autonomic nervous

Criteria for the clinical diagnosis of Metabolic Syndrome

PARAMETER	IDF	NCEP-ATP III	OMS
Abdominal Obesity	Waist circumference 90 cm in men and 80 cm in women (Asia and Latin America)	Waist circumference >102 cm in men + >94 cm in Hispanics >88 cm in women	Waist circumference >90 cm in men and 85 cm in women
High triglycerides	>150 mg/dl	>150 mg/dl	>150 mg/dl
Low cHDL	<40 mg/dl in men <50 mg/dl in women	Low cHDL	<35 mg/dl in men <40 mg/dl in women
Elevated BP	SBP 130 mm/Hg and/or DBP ≥ 85 mm Hg or in antihypertensive treatment	>130/85 mm/Hg	>160/90 mm/Hg
Alteration of the glucose regulation	Fasting blood glucose >100 mg/dl or DM2 previously diagnosed	Fasting blood glucose >100 mg/dL or in treatment/glycemia elevated	Glucose intolerance
Diagnosis	Abdominal Obesity + 2 of the remaining 4 parameters	3 of the 5 parameters	DM, glucose intolerance, altered fasting blood glucose, or demonstrated insulin resistance + 2 of the previous parameters

Fig. 6.2 Diagnostic criteria for metabolic syndrome, according to different associations: **IDF**, *International Diabetes Federation*; **NCEP-ATP III**, *National Cholesterol Education Program's Adult Treatment Panel III*; **WHO**, *World Health Organization.*

system. Furthermore, besides the repercussions on atherosclerosis development, MS and insulin resistance have also been linked to other diseases, such as non-alcoholic fatty liver disease and polycystic ovary syndrome.

6.1.2 Importance of the Microbiota

The **microbiota**, composed of billions of microorganisms, plays a fundamental role in an **individual's metabolic health**. Its importance lies in various aspects.

The microbiota participates in the breakdown of nutrients that the human body cannot digest alone. Additionally, it generates **metabolites** that can influence appetite regulation, glucose metabolism, and lipid synthesis. It has an impact on energy metabolism, regulating body weight and the tendency toward obesity. The microbiota may influence insulin sensitivity and blood sugar regulation, affecting the risk of developing type 2 diabetes. Moreover, the microbiota acts as a key regulator of the immune system, influencing immune response and immune tolerance, as well as modulating the response to certain drugs.

An **imbalance in the microbiota** (dysbiosis) has been associated with metabolic diseases such as metabolic syndrome due to changes in microbial diversity and function (Fig. 6.3).

Nutrition is closely linked to the intestinal microbiota as it can influence the imbalance of bacteria residing in the gut. Therefore, poor dietary habits such as

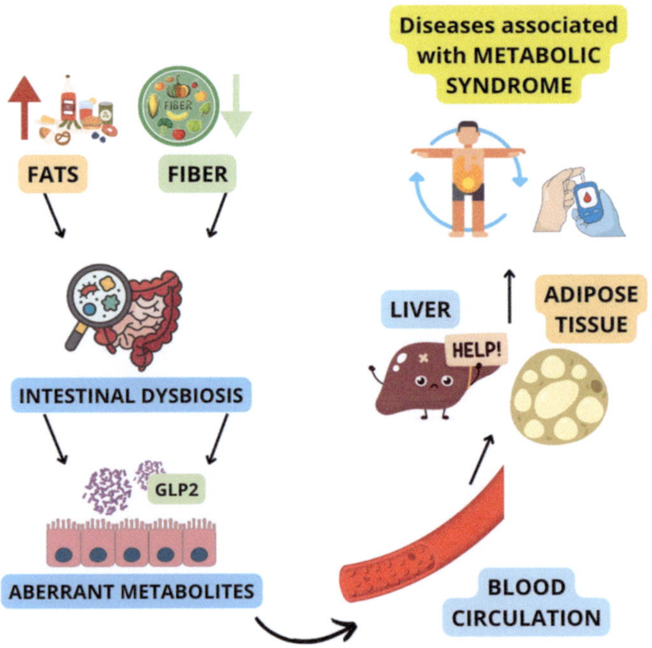

Fig. 6.3 Interaction of the intestinal microbiota and its contribution to metabolic diseases

consuming high-fat, high-sugar, and low-fiber diets will ultimately lead to **intestinal dysbiosis**. This will result in a high concentration of substances that emerge during food breakdown, known as **aberrant metabolites**. These provoke a disruption in the function of **GLP2** (Glucagon-Like Peptide 2). GLP2 is a hormone secreted by endocrine cells in the intestine, especially in response to food intake. It primarily acts in the small intestine, promoting the growth and health of the intestinal mucosa. Additionally, it contributes to the regulation of nutrient absorption and intestinal motility.

With a breakdown in the continuity of the intestinal epithelium, it loses its resistance against **lipopolysaccharides** (LPS), a component of the outer membrane of certain gram-negative bacteria; **trimethylamine** (TMA), an organic compound produced by specific bacteria, and other metabolites that enter circulation, leading to **chronic inflammation** of the liver and adipose tissue, associated with the development of cardiovascular diseases, insulin resistance, and other conditions linked to metabolic syndrome.

Elevated levels of **LPS** in the bloodstream can trigger inflammatory responses, and its chronic presence might contribute to the **chronic inflammation** associated with metabolic diseases. Increased intestinal **permeability** has been suggested to lead to LPS translocation into the bloodstream, triggering systemic responses related to metabolic syndrome.

The liver converts **TMA** into **trimethylamine oxide** (TMAO), a compound linked to fat metabolism, and in some studies, it has been associated with a higher cardiovascular risk. Moreover, research is ongoing regarding how elevated TMAO levels might be associated with metabolic syndrome, although the precise relationship and causality are not yet fully understood.

6.2 Relationship between Intestinal Microbiota and Metabolic Syndrome

6.2.1 Dysbiosis and Disease

The **microorganisms** composing the microbiota are determined by the types of **nutritional sources**. Therefore, dietary characteristics, along with genetic factors, influence the predominance of certain microorganisms over others. The initial microbiota is responsible for generating **metabolites** that can have a beneficial effect on the body, such as anti-inflammatory and antioxidant actions, regulation of intestinal barrier function, as well as the production of vitamins and energy sources.

The intestinal microbiota plays an important role in maintaining individual homeostasis. **Dysbiosis** (changes in the intestinal microbiota and the host's adverse response) is associated with conditions crucial for the development of characteristic alterations of metabolic syndrome.

In individuals with metabolic syndrome, an increase in the ***Firmicutes*/*Bacteroidetes*** ratio has been observed. ***Bifidobacteria*** and ***Bacteroides* spp.** appear to be **protective** against the development of the chronic inflammation characteristic

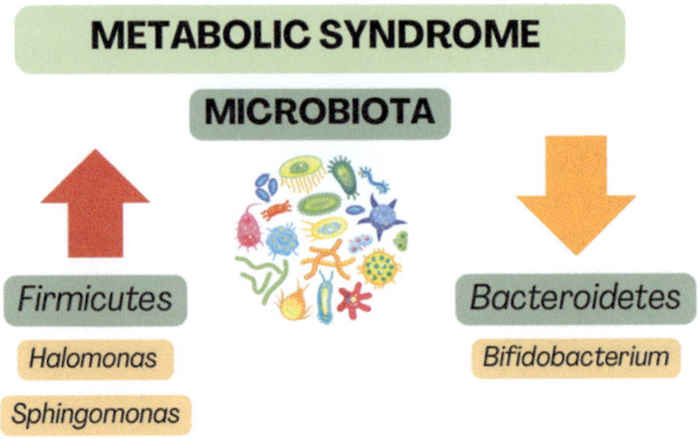

Fig. 6.4 Changes in bacterial species in the microbiota of patients with metabolic syndrome

of MS. It is also asserted that there is a decrease in ***Bifidobacterium*** and an increase in ***Halomonas*** and ***Sphingomonas*** in the intestinal microbiota of patients with metabolic syndrome (Fig. 6.4).

The relationship between **intestinal microbiota** and **metabolic syndrome** is complex and multifaceted. Dysbiosis can trigger a chronic inflammatory response at the intestinal and systemic levels. Moreover, changes in **bacterial composition** can alter the production of **metabolites**, influencing the body's **energy** and metabolic **homeostasis**. An imbalanced microbiota may contribute to increased **intestinal permeability**, allowing the entry of substances that trigger adverse inflammatory and metabolic responses. Consequently, the regulation of adipose tissue and its ability to store fat can be affected, influencing obesity and insulin resistance.

On the other hand, the process of **microbial signaling** involves the transmission of bacterial products from the gut epithelial cells to other organs, shaping critical interactions within the body. **Pattern recognition receptors** (PRRs) like Toll-like receptors (TLRs) and aryl hydrocarbon receptor (AHR) play a pivotal role in recognizing pathogen-associated molecular patterns (PAMPs) present in components like LPS or flagellin, influencing host-microbe immune responses. The AHR, a transcription factor activated by specific bacterial metabolites, such as lactobacilli tryptophan ligand, regulates responses to external stimuli and impacts intestinal motility and metabolism.

Dysbiosis can lead to altered AHR ligand generation, contributing to metabolic disorders and affecting intestinal motility by influencing the enteric neural system. **SCFAs** (short-chain fatty acids), produced through the breakdown of dietary fiber by gut microbes, serve as important signaling molecules by binding to specific receptors (GPR43 and GPR41), triggering the secretion of GLP-1 from L-cells. This **GLP-1** impacts insulin release and appetite regulation, while **SCFAs** themselves play a crucial role in gluconeogenesis and overall gastrointestinal health.

The **interconnectedness** of microbial metabolites, particularly SCFAs, and their interactions with receptors in the gut underline their significance in regulating gastrointestinal motility and metabolic function. Modulating these interactions through changes in the gut microbiome could potentially offer novel therapeutic avenues for metabolic diseases.

6.3 Mechanisms of Association

Currently, there are studies that have shown changes in bacterial composition in individuals with metabolic syndrome, identifying significant bacteria in terms of diversity and types of bacteria present.

6.3.1 Probiotics and Prebiotics

Clinical trials have been conducted to assess the impact of **probiotics and prebiotics** on modulating the microbiota and improving metabolic parameters in individuals with this syndrome (Fig. 6.5).

Prebiotics, such as inulin and fructo-oligosaccharides, may promote the growth of beneficial bacteria in the gut, thereby improving microbial diversity. Moreover, studies suggest that prebiotics could have beneficial effects on regulating metabolic parameters, such as glycemia, insulin sensitivity, and reducing inflammation in people with metabolic syndrome (MS). **Probiotics** also have the ability to alter the composition of the gut microbiota by increasing the presence of beneficial strains.

	PROBIOTICS	PREBIOTICS
Definition	Live microorganisms, typically beneficial bacteria, that, when consumed in adequate amounts, confer health benefits.	Non-digestible compounds that act as food for beneficial bacteria in the gut, promoting their growth and activity.
Function	They colonize the gastrointestinal tract and are believed to improve the balance of the gut microbiota by increasing the presence of beneficial bacteria.	They are not live organisms but rather dietary components that selectively encourage the growth of beneficial bacteria already present in the gut.
Common sources	Yogurts, certain fermented milk products, dietary supplements, and various fermented foods. Ex. *Lactobacillus, Bifidobacterium, certain strains of Streptococcus, and Saccharomyces boulardii.*	Some fiber-rich foods such as garlic, onions, bananas, asparagus, leeks, and certain types of cereals and legumes.
Examples	Probiotics are thought to improve digestion, strengthen the immune system, aid in nutrient absorption, and possibly reduce inflammation.	They help to feed and stimulate the growth of beneficial bacteria in the gut, which can improve gut health, nutrient absorption, and promote a healthy balance of the microbiota.

Fig. 6.5 Differences between probiotics and prebiotics

Research suggests that probiotics might have positive effects on obesity, insulin resistance, type 2 diabetes, and cardiovascular health. However, outcomes vary as they depend on the specific strains used.

Clinical studies have evaluated the effects of prebiotics and probiotics in different population groups, from adults with MS to children at risk of obesity. Additionally, the effects of combinations of probiotics and prebiotics have been studied, as well as their **synergy** with other treatments or lifestyle changes aimed at improving metabolic health. Despite advancements, challenges exist due to the **heterogeneity** of responses, as there is **variability** in individual responses to these compounds. This has led to exploring the influence of genetics, diet, and other factors that may modulate efficacy. Some studies conclude that *prebiotic* consumption affects/modifies **anthropometric variables**, while *probiotic* intake impacts **biochemical variables**. Concerning the risk/presence of MS, probiotic consumption seems to have a more significant protective influence than prebiotic consumption. Furthermore, studies are being conducted to identify **optimal doses** and **treatment duration** to achieve consistent metabolic benefits.

6.3.2 Fecal Transplantation

Several studies have investigated **fecal microbiota transplantation** (FMT) as a strategy to modify bacterial composition and improve metabolic health in patients with metabolic diseases. Currently, fecal microbiota transplantation involves transferring stool from a healthy donor to another patient with the aim of changing or restoring their microbiota's composition and function. Its only accepted clinical application at present is in the treatment of recurrent ***Clostridium difficile*** infection. Nevertheless, its use is being studied in diseases such as **inflammatory bowel disease**, **autism**, and **metabolic disorders**. Within this latter group, we find metabolic syndrome, obesity, and type 2 diabetes, all characterized by dysbiosis of the gut microbiota. However, results from studies on fecal transplantation and metabolic syndrome have been variable thus far. Some show potential improvements in insulin sensitivity and body composition, while others do not find significant effects.

Advancements in clinical studies and research have provided valuable insights into how the **gut microbiota** influences the development and progression of metabolic syndrome, although further research is needed to fully understand these mechanisms and develop precise therapeutic strategies.

6.4 Therapeutic Strategies and Future

6.4.1 Emerging Therapies

Emerging therapies to address metabolic syndrome focus on various areas, from modulating the microbiota to utilizing **gene therapies**.

Currently, as mentioned earlier, efforts revolve around modulating the microbiota through prebiotics and probiotics, as well as fecal microbiota transplantation (FMT). However, **pharmacological therapies** also exist, aiming to modulate metabolism through drugs. These target specific lipid, glucose, and other components related to MS. Research is focused on molecules aiming to reduce insulin resistance, control inflammation, and improve insulin sensitivity.

Non-pharmacological therapies place great emphasis on regular physical exercise and **lifestyle** changes. There's also a developing area in **gene therapy**. Approaches are being explored to genetically modify cells to influence metabolism and address specific aspects of MS.

6.4.2 Challenges and Future Directions

The aim is to achieve **treatment personalization**, identifying personalized therapeutic approaches based on **genetics**, individual **microbiota**, and other factors. As new therapies are developed, assessing their long-term safety and effectiveness in different patient subgroups is essential.

It is crucial to highlight that addressing metabolic syndrome requires a **combination** of pharmacological therapies, lifestyle changes, and holistic approaches to achieve optimal results. Understanding the **complex metabolic interactions** and **biological individuality** is critical for advancing metabolic syndrome treatment.

6.5 Conclusion

Metabolic syndrome, a complex health concern, intertwines metabolic dysregulations with chronic inflammation and insulin resistance.

The **microbiota** emerges as a **pivotal player**, impacting nutrient breakdown, metabolite generation, and immune modulation. Disruptions in this delicate balance, termed dysbiosis, closely associate with metabolic diseases, influencing microbial diversity and function.

Various interventions, such as probiotics, prebiotics, and fecal transplantation, have been explored for their potential in restoring microbial balance and improving metabolic parameters. While promising, these strategies face challenges in consistency and individual responses.

Personalized therapeutic approaches, integrating genetics, microbiota analysis, and multifaceted treatments, represent the future direction for tackling metabolic syndrome effectively. These insights pave the way for a holistic understanding, emphasizing the need to intertwine genetics, lifestyle modifications, and innovative therapies to combat metabolic syndrome comprehensively.

Suggested Readings

1. Raghubeer S. The influence of epigenetics and inflammation on cardiometabolic risks. Semin Cell Dev Biol. 2024;154(Pt C):175–84.
2. Kuckuck S, Lengton R, Boon MR, Boersma E, Penninx BWJH, Kavousi M, van Rossum EFC. Long-term glucocorticoids in relation to the metabolic syndrome and cardiovascular disease: A systematic review and meta-analysis. J Intern Med. 2024;295(1):2–19.
3. Codazzi V, Frontino G, Galimberti L, Giustina A, Petrelli A. Mechanisms and risk factors of metabolic syndrome in children and adolescents. Endocrine. 2024;84(1):16–28. https://doi.org/10.1007/s12020-023-03642-x.
4. Christian Flemming GM. Definition and early diagnosis of metabolic syndrome in children. J Pediatr Endocrinol Metab. 2020;33(7):821–33.
5. Corro AC, Matheus NJ, Medina CE. Microbiota intestinal y su relación con trastornos metabólicos. Rev Venezol Salud Púb. 2016;4(2):41–4.
6. Milian EJ, Anzueles JB, Betancourt-Castellanos L, Izaguirre-Bordelois M, Caballero AE. Síndrome metabólico y su relación con la microbiota intestinal. Repert Med Cir. 2024;33(1):14–20. https://doi.org/10.31260/RepertMedCir.01217372
7. Correa ML. Prebiotics and probiotics consumption in relation to metabolic syndrome markers in university students. Nutr Clinica Diet Hosp. 2019;39:171–82.
8. Portincasa P, Khalil M, Graziani A, Frühbeck G, Baffy G, Garruti G, et al. Gut microbes in metabolic disturbances. Promising role for therapeutic manipulations? Eur J Intern Med. 2023;119:13–30.
9. Ambroselli D, Masciulli F, Romano E, Catanzaro G, Besharat ZM, Massari MC, et al. New advances in metabolic syndrome, from prevention to treatment: the role of diet and food. Nutrients. 2023;15(3):640.
10. Malnick SDH, Fisher D, Somin M, Neuman MG. Treating the metabolic syndrome by fecal transplantation—current status. Biology. 2021;10:447.

Microbiota and the Cardiovascular System

7

Óscar Lorenzo, Jairo Lumpuy-Castillo, Cristina Espadas, Octavian Parascinet, and Sacramento Martínez-Albaladejo

7.1 Cardiovascular Disease as Main Cause of Worldwide Morbimortality

According to the World Health Organization (https://www.who.int), cardiovascular diseases (CVD) cause the deaths of 17.9 million people per year, corresponding to 31% of all deaths. CVD include a range of disorders affecting the heart and blood vessels. The most common types of CVD include coronary artery disease (CAD), heart failure (HF), stroke, and myocardial infarct. Remarkedly, several risk factors contribute to the development of CVD. These include advanced age, diabetes, obesity, dyslipidemia, and hypertension but also smoking habit, sedentary lifestyle, and unhealthy diets [1]. Given the significant impact of CVD on public health, efforts to reduce their prevalence and improve outcomes involve a combination of population-wide interventions and individual healthcare. In this sense, early detection of CVD, adherence to pharmacological treatments, and the effective management of associated risk factors and lifestyle modifications remain crucial in the global fight against CVD [2].

7.2 Therapeutic Interventions for Cardiovascular Diseases

For pharmacological interventions, the choice and dosage of drugs may depend on the specific cardiovascular condition, presence of comorbidities, and patient characteristics. Mainly, statins lower cholesterol levels by inhibition of cholesterol synthesis in the liver, reducing the risk of atherosclerosis and cardiovascular events [3, 4]. Beta-blockers lessen the effects of adrenaline on the heart, reducing heart rate and

Ó. Lorenzo (✉) · J. Lumpuy-Castillo · C. Espadas · O. Parascinet · S. Martínez-Albaladejo
Laboratory of Diabetes and Vascular pathology, IIS-Fundación Jiménez Díaz, Medicine Department, CIBERDEM, Universidad Autónoma, Madrid, Spain
e-mail: OLorenzo@fjd.es

J. Ruiz-Tovar (ed.), *Dysbiosis*, https://doi.org/10.1007/978-3-031-65650-7_7

blood pressure during hypertension, angina, and HF. Mineralocorticoid receptor antagonists (MRAs) attenuate the effects of mineralocorticoid hormones, playing a key role in regulating electrolytes such as sodium and potassium. Antihypertensive drugs, such as Angiotensin-Converting Enzyme (ACE) Inhibitors, can reduce blood pressure by blocking the conversion of angiotensin I to angiotensin II. Angiotensin II Receptor Blockers (ARBs) also attenuate the effects of angiotensin II leading to vasodilation and reduced blood pressure. Calcium Channel Blockers relax blood vessels and decrease the heart's workload and blood pressure, while diuretics eliminate excess of salt and water from the body, reducing blood volume and hypertension. Other medications, such as anticoagulants and antiplatelets, prevent blood clot formation, whereas antiarrhythmics control abnormal heart rhythms [3, 4]. Nitroglycerin and other vasodilators relax blood vessels and relieve angina symptoms, lessening blood pressure and heart workload.

However, efficacy of these cardiovascular therapies can vary among individuals with different age and sex, and not all patients optimally respond to the same treatments [5, 6]. Delays in diagnosis and treatment initiation can also result in disease progression, affecting the effectiveness of interventions. Also, CVD are often complex and multifactorial, and the presence of comorbidities, such as diabetes, hypertension, or kidney disease, can worsen prognosis. Drug interactions may also affect the efficacy and safety of these therapies, and some patients develop resistance or tolerance to certain medications (i.e., statin) over time. Moreover, a lack of adherence to prescribed medications is a common issue, and a limited access to medications in some cases can hinder drug administration [7]. Finally, environmental factors such as nutrition and the intestinal microbiota should be considered for the CVD treatment [8].

7.3 Microbiota and the Cardiovascular System

The microbiota refers to the community of microorganisms, including bacteria, viruses, fungi, and archaea, that inhabit the human body. Trillions of microorganisms residing in the gastrointestinal tract influence cardiovascular health [9]. Gut microbiota plays a role in the metabolism of dietary compounds, including sugar, lipids, and proteins, and may regulate the metabolic, immune, endocrine, and cardiovascular systems by the release of metabolites. The distribution of microbes is relatively stable, with consistency among family members but inconsistency among unrelated individuals from different geographies. A healthy microbiota consists of adequate balance of four groups of bacteria, namely, *Actinobacteria*, *Firmicutes*, *Proteobacteria*, and *Bacteroides*, which continuously adapt to lifestyle changes [10]. Interestingly, a bidirectional communication between gut microbiota and extra-intestinal organs like heart (gut-heart axis) has been intensively studied during the last two decades.

In this sense, variations in the gut microbiota (higher *Firmicutes/Bacteroidetes* ratio) were found in individuals with CAD [11]. Other authors described a lower relative abundance of *Roseburia* and *Eubacterium* in these patients [12]. Also, preliminary clinical research uncovered microbiota alterations among individuals with HF. These disruptions in microbial communities can result from the intestinal hypoperfusion that leads to changes in local pH and gut luminal hypoxia [13]. Also, an adaptive re-distribution of the systemic circulation to the intestine, as a consequence of a decreased cardiac output, influences on microbiota composition [14]. Thus, intestinal wall edema and wall thickening may increase intestinal permeability, facilitating the passage of bacteria and endotoxins (i.e., lipopolysaccharides, LPS) to the systemic bloodstream [15]. In addition, a link between the composition and distribution of the gut microbiota has been related with the cardiovascular function. Imbalances in the gut microbiota (dysbiosis) or in derived metabolites might contribute to the development of CVD [16]. Dysbiosis promoted gut permeability and endotoxemia that activate immune responses and systemic inflammation [17]. It can also reduce gut-derived cardioprotective metabolites and contribute to disturbances in glucose and lipid metabolism, potentially increasing CVD [18]. Dysbiosis also influenced the production of bioactive compounds that alter endothelial function and blood pressure and affect coagulation factors and platelet aggregation, leading to hemostatic pathologies [19]. Finally, dysbiosis encouraged maladaptive cardiac remodeling, which may provoke HF [20].

7.4 Microbiota-Derived Metabolites

Many gut bacteria contribute positively to cardiovascular health, but other species produce toxic metabolites or by-products with potential adverse actions. These effects can vary depending on the overall composition of the microbiota, host genetics, and environmental agents. Also, some metabolites may trigger dual roles, acting as signaling molecules or contributors to both health and disease depending on context [21].

The short-chain fatty acids (SCFAs), acetate, propionate, and butyrate, are produced by fermentation of dietary fibers by gut bacteria. SCFAs contribute to the maintenance of the intestinal epithelial barrier, which helps to prevent the entry of harmful substances and pathogens from the gut lumen into the bloodstream [22]. They also stimulate the production of mucus by goblet cells as a protective layer to trap and remove potentially toxic agents and contribute to the maintenance of a slightly acidic environment in the colon to inhibit the growth of undesirable bacteria. SCFAs activate regulatory T cells improving immune tolerance and prevention of inappropriate responses against the gut microbiota or dietary antigens [23]. SCFAs, particularly propionate, regulate appetite and metabolism by release of intestinal hormones [24]. In turn, butyrate induces anti-inflammatory outcomes and can be used as an important energy source for colonocytes (cells lining the colon). Also, butyrate prompts apoptosis in abnormal cells (i.e., cancer cells) [25]. Other gut-derived antioxidant and anti-inflammatory metabolites are synthesized from polyphenols from fruits and vegetables [26]. Other bacteria convert linoleic acid into conjugated linoleic acid (CLA) with anti-inflammatory and anti-cancer properties [27]. Moreover, gut-derived vitamins, including B vitamins (B12, folate) and vitamin K, are essential for energy metabolism and blood clotting [28]. Interestingly, absorption of certain vitamins and minerals is favored by SCFA production [29]. Finally, fermentation-derived gases including hydrogen gas (H_2), methane (CH_4), and carbon dioxide (CO_2) may exhibit signaling functions on gut motility and nutrient adsorption [30]. Also, hydrogen sulfide (H_2S), produced from amino acid degradation, can induce vasodilatory, anti-inflammatory, and antioxidant effects [31].

In contrast, certain bacteria produce unfavorable molecules. They can metabolize dietary compounds like choline and L-carnitine to trimethylamine (TMA), which is absorbed into the bloodstream and further oxidize in the liver to form the uremic toxin, trimethylamine *N*-oxide (TMAO). Elevated levels of TMAO induced inflammation and endothelial dysfunction, favoring development of atherosclerotic plaques [32]. It also upregulated the expression of genes involved in cholesterol absorption and transport and enhanced cholesterol accumulation in macrophages to generate foam cells [33]. Other bacteria produce indole as a by-product of tryptophan metabolism. Indole is further metabolized in the liver to form another uremic toxin, indoxyl sulfate, which has pro-inflammatory and pro-oxidative actions. Importantly, indoxyl sulfate has been implicated in the progression of a main cardiovascular comorbidity, the chronic kidney disease (CKD) [34]. Ammonia (NH_3) is also a toxic compound that can be produced from dietary proteins by bacteria. Elevated levels of ammonia in the bloodstream triggered systemic effects (liver, kidney) that indirectly impacted on cardiovascular health [35]. It also interfered with nitric oxide production and availability, affecting blood vessel function. Furthermore, excessive production of SCFAs like propionate may lead to insulin resistance and metabolic disturbances [36], and high levels of H_2S can induce ulcerative colitis and inflammatory bowel disease [37].

7.5 Microbiota and Cardiovascular Risk Factors

7.5.1 Dyslipidemia and Obesity

The relationship between the gut microbiota and obesity is complex and influenced by genetics, diet, lifestyle, and environmental exposures. High-fat diets and those low in fiber have been associated with dysbiosis, whereas diets rich in plant-based foods and fiber promote the growth of beneficial bacteria [38]. Many studies have observed differences in the microbiota composition and distribution between obese and non-obese individuals. Dysbiosis can modify the extraction of energy from the diet and the storage of calories in the body [39]. It may impact on SCFA production, energy balance, and gut permeability. In turn, metabolic endotoxemia can trigger inflammation and metabolic disorders such as obesity [40]. Moreover, dysbiosis may disrupt communication with the host's central nervous system influencing appetite control [41]. Also, gut bacteria can modify various enzymatic activities for conversion of primary bile acids into secondary bile acids, playing a crucial role in the digestion and absorption of dietary fats [42]. Thus, SCFAs-producing bacteria can lower cholesterol absorption, while those bacteria producing TMAO or LPS damage liver and hepatic lipid metabolism, contributing to obesity and development of non-alcoholic fatty liver disease (NAFLD) [43]. In this line, composition of gut microbiota influence on adipose tissue function by regulating secretion of adipokines and hormones like leptin and adiponectin related to appetite and insulin sensitivity [44]. Both NAFLD and CVD share common pathophysiological mechanisms, including oxidative stress, inflammation, and alterations in lipid metabolism. Thus, cardiac dysfunction is commonly observed in individuals with NAFLD [45].

However, probiotics have the potential to alleviate lipid abnormalities in overweight or obese adults [46]. *Lactobacillus* and *Bifidobacterium* genera are the two most used probiotics strains. Some studies, mainly in animals, have reported that lactic acid bacteria can prevent and improve obesity by regulating the gut microecological balance, promoting lipid metabolism, and reducing serum lipid levels. Probiotic consumption markedly decreased the plasma levels of total cholesterol, triglycerides, and LDL-C [46]. This effect could be mirrored in non-obese healthy adults with hyperlipidemia [47], suggesting a direct anti-hyperlipidemic effect of specific bacteria. In this sense, single probiotics, especially *Lactobacillus*, showed a potential benefit on obesity and dyslipidemia [48]. However, some probiotic supplementation did not increase HDL levels neither the HDL/LDL ratio [49]. In a similar way, prebiotics and synbiotics (mixtures of probiotics and prebiotics) also worked as adjuvant therapy against dyslipidemia [50]. Most of the prebiotics used such as inulin, fructo-oligosaccharides, dietary fiber, and gums are derived from plants. In particular, poly-D-3-hydroxybutyric acid favored the growth of beneficial microbiota and attenuated the obesity-associated dyslipidemia [51].

7.5.2 Glycemia and Insulin Resistance

The intricate interactions between the microbiota and the host can influence various aspects of glucose homeostasis, including inflammation and insulin sensitivity [52]. Dysbiosis produces chronic low-grade inflammation, which impairs glucose metabolism. In this sense, the release of bacterial metabolites such as butyrate, secondary bile acids, and polyphenol-derived agents correlated with an improved insulin sensitivity and glucose homeostasis [53]. Bile acids interacted with the farnesoid X receptor (FXR) to release fibroblast growth factor 19 (FGF19), which regulate bile acid production and liver gluconeogenesis [54]. Bile acids also activated the Takeda G protein-coupled receptor 5 (TGR5) TGR5 to stimulate gut hormones like glucagon-like peptide-1 (GLP-1) synthesis [55]. Moreover, specific bacteria affected secretion of GLP-1 and peptide YY (PYY) that reduce appetite and insulin secretion [56].

In this case, some probiotic- and prebiotic-derived improvements have been also reported on glucose metabolism. In a systematic review, 27 probiotic interventions (*Lactobacillus*, *Bifidobacterium*, *Clostridium*, and *Akkermansia*) in animals triggered favorable actions on insulin resistance. However, in seven clinical trials, five of them showed benefits in insulin resistance, but two others demonstrated no effects [57]. In another meta-analysis, probiotics improved glucose metabolism by a modest degree, with a greater result when multiple species of probiotics were administrated [58]. Also, probiotics reduced HbA1c (and the lipid profile) in patients with prediabetes [59] and in those with gestational diabetes [60]. In addition, increasing evidence demonstrated that prebiotics could lead to clinical advantages for glycemic control [61]. However, it is not clear whether these effects can be due to modification of the microbiota or through increasing substrate availability for fermentation.

7.6 Microbiota and Cardiovascular Comorbidities

Gut dysbiosis can be a causative insult leading to diabetes, sustained increase in blood pressure, and CKD, but also, these comorbidities may impact the microbiome to an extent that the altered microbiota contributes to the progression and/or continued pathological states.

7.6.1 Diabetes

Research in the field of dysbiosis and both type 1 diabetes (T1D) and type 2 diabetes (T2D) are progressing. However, the specific mechanisms and causal relationships are still unknown [62]. Early-life dysbiosis may influence the risk of developing T1D in children. Some research suggests a potential link between certain viruses in the gut and the development of T1D [63]. Also, reduction of microbial diversity has been described in both individuals with T1D and T2D [62], and especially alterations in bile acid metabolism have been associated with T2D development [64]. Dysbiosis may reshape intestinal barrier functions and host metabolic and signaling pathways that are directly or indirectly related to the insulin resistance in T2D. It also causes dyslipidemia and triglyceridemia. A perturbed *Bacteroidetes/Firmicutes* ratio has been linked with increased intestinal permeability, with infiltration of bacteria by-products through a leaky gut barrier triggering subsequent inflammatory responses characteristic of diabetes [65].

Nevertheless, as stated before, probiotics and prebiotics supplementation has been efficient for lipid and glucose metabolism, which has improved T1D and T2D evolution in both human and animal models [66, 67]. Children with newly diagnosed T1D managed with standard treatment along with probiotics showed better glycemic control and a decrease in insulin requirements [68]. Also, a significant enhancement in the HOMA-IR, HbA1c, and fasting blood glucose levels was described after probiotic intervention in T2D patients [69]. Particularly, higher abundance of the anti-inflammatory and mucin/SCFAs-producer *Akkermansia muciniphila* was associated with positive metabolic parameters and a reduced risk of T2D [70].

In addition, prebiotics and synbiotics have lessened insulin resistance [50], and the clinical use of supplemented fibers (i.e., oligofructose) with hypoglycemic medications might mitigate early stages of T2D [71].

7.6.2 Hypertension

Changes in the composition and diversity of gut bacteria have been also observed in individuals with hypertension [72]. The gut microbiota interacts with the immune system, and immune responses may influence blood pressure regulation. Also, low-grade inflammation has been recognized as a main trigger of hypertension in human [73]. In this line, dysbiosis is associated with hypertension in patients and in several preclinical models. Dysbiosis can regulate salt sensitivity by affecting sodium and water balance by activation of the renin-angiotensin system [74]. It can increase sympathetic tone and systemic inflammation while decreasing mesenteric blood flow [75]. Some bacteria are also involved in the conversion of dietary nitrates into nitric oxide (NO), which promote blood vessel dilation [76]. Especially butyrate promotes to vasodilation [77]. In contrast, TMAO was associated with hypertension development [78].

A recent meta-analysis suggested that probiotics supplementation could be used as a complementary therapy for controlling high blood pressure [79]. Probiotics were efficient in declining both systolic and diastolic blood pressure. *Lactobacillus* and *Bifidobacterium* may synthesize neurotransmitters, SCFAs, and antioxidant factors that may be responsible of vessel relaxation [80]. Although controversial findings are raised, positive outcomes from both in vitro and in vivo studies have suggested the need for further evaluation of the antihypertensive properties of prebiotics. A recent meta-analysis of five trials indicated that supplementation with inulin did not reduce either systolic or diastolic blood pressure. However, prebiotic fiber contributed to the anti-hypertensive actions of oats by increasing gamma-aminobutyric acid (GABA) levels [81].

7.6.3 Chronic Kidney Disease

The association between the intestine and kidneys is termed the gut-kidney axis. The immune disturbance in gut dysbiosis causes the abnormal proliferation and differentiation of lymphocytes, leading to the production of autoantibodies associated with CKD [82]. Gut bacteria produce uremic toxins or protein-bound uremic toxins, mainly indoxyl sulfate, *p*-cresyl sulfate, hippuric acid, TMAO, asymmetric dimethylarginine (ADMA), and cytokines TNF-α and IL-6 [83]. Dysbiosis also causes neuroendocrine dysfunction, which can aggravate CKD and its cardiovascular complications [84], and impairs the energy supply to the colonic epithelium promoting epithelial permeability and a leaky gut [85]. In this scenario, chronic inflammation was also linked to CKD [86], and circulating LPS and bacterial DNA favored CKD and its associated mortality [87].

However, probiotic administration may induce also potential benefits in improving symptoms and quality of life, reducing inflammation, and delaying the progression of kidney failure. Most randomized controlled trials on probiotic treatment were focused on advanced stages (3–5) of CKD (hemodialysis, peritoneal dialysis), but probiotics decreased plasma concentrations of uremic toxins, inflammation, and gastrointestinal symptoms [88]. Again, *Lactobacillus* slowed CKD progression by increasing availability of SCFAs with anti-inflammatory properties [89]. Nevertheless, a recent metanalysis concluded that it is uncertain whether probiotics, prebiotics, or synbiotics can improve eGFR, proteinuria, and uremic toxins after CKD [88].

7.7 Cardiovascular Pharmacology and Microbiota

A key point should consider whether microbiota can influence cardiovascular medications and if these drugs can affect microbiota composition. Gut bacteria may produce enzymes involved in oral drugs metabolism (acetylation, β-glucuronidation, deconjugation, dihydroxylation, denitration, hydrolysis, reduction) disturbing their absorption across the gut and through the bloodstream [90]. Also, microbiota may inactivate specific medications or alter their pharmacokinetics by known or unknown mechanisms. Specific bacteria reduced amount of statins reaching target tissues and changed the linked FXR signaling [91]. An antibiotic treatment increased bioavailability of a calcium channel blocker [92], and some strains of *Eggerthella lenta* were responsible for converting digoxin into an inactive metabolites [93]. On the other hand, hypercholesterolemic subjects treated with atorvastatin presented an increased level of anti-inflammatory gut bacteria such as *Faecalibacterium prausnitzii* and *Akkermansia muciniphila* and other bacteria involved in bile acid metabolism [94]. ACE inhibitors induced beneficial effects on hypertensive rats by diminishing gut dysbiosis and ameliorating the intestinal permeability [90]. In turn, ARBs were able to normalize the *Firmicutes*/*Bacteroidetes* ratio in HF patients [95], and inhibitors of platelet aggregation induced positive variations of *Ruminococcaceae*, *Prevotella*, *Barnesiella,* and *Bacteroides* [96]. Therefore, microbiota can metabolize cardiovascular drugs which results in altered pharmacokinetics and pharmacodynamics or formation of toxic metabolites which may interfere with drug responses, but also main cardiovascular medications could unbalance the growing of specific gut bacteria.

7.8 Conclusion

The bidirectional relationship between gut microbiota and the cardiovascular system is an evolving area of research. There is growing evidence supporting a connection between specific bacteria strains with cardiovascular risk factors and comorbidities. Understanding the complex interplay between bacteria with host immune responses and glucose/lipid metabolism may suggest new therapeutic interventions. Manipulating the composition and distribution of microbiota and of derived metabolites (i.e., SCFAs, bile acids and vitamins, and TMA, ammonia, and uremic toxins) through specific probiotics (e.g., *Lactobacillus*, *Bifidobacteria*, *Verrucomicrobia*) may hold promise for establishing a microbial balance in the gut. Undoubtedly, these approaches should complement the actions of specific diets (or prebiotics) and medication in each patient. However, there is still no standard in the dosage and duration of the use of probiotics, neither its potential interactions with drugs against CVD or associated comorbidities, such as statins, anti-hypertensives, anti-coagulants, or anti-diabetics.

References

1. Global Cardiovascular Risk Consortium, Magnussen C, Ojeda FM, et al. Global effect of modifiable risk factors on cardiovascular disease and mortality. N Engl J Med. 2023;389:1273–85. https://doi.org/10.1056/NEJMoa2206916.
2. Ghodeshwar GK, Dube A, Khobragade D. Impact of lifestyle modifications on cardiovascular health: a narrative review. Cureus. 2023;15:e42616. https://doi.org/10.7759/cureus.42616.
3. McDonagh TA, Metra M, Adamo M, et al. 2023 focused update of the 2021 ESC guidelines for the diagnosis and treatment of acute and chronic heart failure. Eur Heart J. 2023;44:3627–39. https://doi.org/10.1093/eurheartj/ehad195.
4. Heidenreich PA, Bozkurt B, Aguilar D, Allen LA, Byun JJ, Colvin MM, Deswal A, Drazner MH, Dunlay SM, Evers LR, Fang JC. 2022 AHA/ACC/HFSA guideline for the management of heart failure: a report of the American College of Cardiology/American Heart Association Joint Committee on Clinical Practice Guidelines. Circulation. 2022.; https://www.ahajournals.org/doi/full/10.1161/CIR.0000000000001063. Accessed 28 Dec 2023.
5. Lima Dos Santos CC, Matharoo AS, Pinzón Cueva E, et al. The influence of sex, age, and race on coronary artery disease: a narrative review. Cureus. 2023;15:e47799. https://doi.org/10.7759/cureus.47799.
6. Regitz-Zagrosek V, Gebhard C. Gender medicine: effects of sex and gender on cardiovascular disease manifestation and outcomes. Nat Rev Cardiol. 2023;20:236–47. https://doi.org/10.1038/s41569-022-00797-4.
7. Khunti K, Danese MD, Kutikova L, et al. Association of a combined measure of adherence and treatment intensity with cardiovascular outcomes in patients with atherosclerosis or other cardiovascular risk factors treated with statins and/or ezetimibe. JAMA Netw Open. 2018;1:e185554. https://doi.org/10.1001/jamanetworkopen.2018.5554.
8. Tyrovola D, Soulaidopoulos S, Tsioufis C, Lazaros G. The role of nutrition in cardiovascular disease: current concepts and trends. Nutrients. 2023;15:1064. https://doi.org/10.3390/nu15051064.
9. Ogunrinola GA, Oyewale JO, Oshamika OO, Olasehinde GI. The human microbiome and its impacts on health. Int J Microbiol. 2020;2020:8045646. https://doi.org/10.1155/2020/8045646.
10. Rinninella E, Raoul P, Cintoni M, et al. What is the healthy gut microbiota composition? A changing ecosystem across age, environment, diet, and diseases. Microorganisms. 2019;7:14. https://doi.org/10.3390/microorganisms7010014.
11. Cui L, Zhao T, Hu H, et al. Association study of gut Flora in coronary heart disease through high-throughput sequencing. Biomed Res Int. 2017;2017:e3796359. https://doi.org/10.1155/2017/3796359.
12. Karlsson FH, Fåk F, Nookaew I, et al. Symptomatic atherosclerosis is associated with an altered gut metagenome. Nat Commun. 2012;3:1245. https://doi.org/10.1038/ncomms2266.
13. Gallo A, Macerola N, Favuzzi AM, et al. The gut in heart failure: current knowledge and novel frontiers. Med Princ Pract Int J Kuwait Univ Health Sci Cent. 2022;31:203–14. https://doi.org/10.1159/000522284.
14. Tang WHW, Li DY, Hazen SL. Dietary metabolism, the gut microbiome, and heart failure. Nat Rev Cardiol. 2019;16:137–54. https://doi.org/10.1038/s41569-018-0108-7.
15. Sandek A, Bauditz J, Swidsinski A, et al. Altered intestinal function in patients with chronic heart failure. J Am Coll Cardiol. 2007;50:1561–9. https://doi.org/10.1016/j.jacc.2007.07.016.

16. Xu H, Wang X, Feng W, et al. The gut microbiota and its interactions with cardiovascular disease. Microb Biotechnol. 2020;13:637–56. https://doi.org/10.1111/1751-7915.13524.
17. Violi F, Cammisotto V, Bartimoccia S, et al. Gut-derived low-grade endotoxaemia, atherothrombosis and cardiovascular disease. Nat Rev Cardiol. 2023;20:24–37. https://doi.org/10.1038/s41569-022-00737-2.
18. Duttaroy AK. Role of gut microbiota and their metabolites on atherosclerosis, hypertension and human blood platelet function: a review. Nutrients. 2021;13:144. https://doi.org/10.3390/nu13010144.
19. Maiuolo J, Carresi C, Gliozzi M, et al. The contribution of gut microbiota and endothelial dysfunction in the development of arterial hypertension in animal models and in humans. Int J Mol Sci. 2022;23:3698. https://doi.org/10.3390/ijms23073698.
20. Masenga SK, Povia JP, Lwiindi PC, Kirabo A. Recent advances in microbiota-associated metabolites in heart failure. Biomedicines. 2023;11:2313. https://doi.org/10.3390/biomedicines11082313.
21. Zhang Y, Chen R, Zhang D, et al. Metabolite interactions between host and microbiota during health and disease: which feeds the other? Biomed Pharmacother. 2023;160:114295. https://doi.org/10.1016/j.biopha.2023.114295.
22. Pérez-Reytor D, Puebla C, Karahanian E, García K. Use of short-chain fatty acids for the recovery of the intestinal epithelial barrier affected by bacterial toxins. Front Physiol. 2021;12:650313. https://doi.org/10.3389/fphys.2021.650313.
23. Kim CH, Park J, Kim M. Gut microbiota-derived short-chain fatty acids, T cells, and inflammation. Immune Netw. 2014;14:277–88. https://doi.org/10.4110/in.2014.14.6.277.
24. Zhang Y, Li X, Huang G, et al. Propionate stimulates the secretion of satiety hormones and reduces acute appetite in a cecal fistula pig model. Anim Nutr. 2022;10:390–8. https://doi.org/10.1016/j.aninu.2022.06.003.
25. Salvi PS, Cowles RA. Butyrate and the intestinal epithelium: modulation of proliferation and inflammation in homeostasis and disease. Cells. 2021;10:1775. https://doi.org/10.3390/cells10071775.
26. Wang X, Qi Y, Zheng H. Dietary polyphenol, gut microbiota, and health benefits. Antioxidants. 2022;11:1212. https://doi.org/10.3390/antiox11061212.
27. Nasrollahzadeh A, Mollaei Tavani S, Arjeh E, Jafari SM. Production of conjugated linoleic acid by lactic acid bacteria; important factors and optimum conditions. Food Chem X. 2023;20:100942. https://doi.org/10.1016/j.fochx.2023.100942.
28. Gholami H, Chmiel JA, Burton JP, Maleki Vareki S. The role of microbiota-derived vitamins in immune homeostasis and enhancing cancer immunotherapy. Cancers. 2023;15:1300. https://doi.org/10.3390/cancers15041300.
29. den Besten G, van Eunen K, Groen AK, et al. The role of short-chain fatty acids in the interplay between diet, gut microbiota, and host energy metabolism. J Lipid Res. 2013;54:2325–40. https://doi.org/10.1194/jlr.R036012.
30. González-Tenorio D, Muñoz-Páez KM, Buitrón G, Valdez-Vazquez I. Fermentation of organic wastes and CO2 + H2 off-gas by microbiotas provides short-chain fatty acids and ethanol for n-caproate production. J CO2 Util. 2020;42:101314. https://doi.org/10.1016/j.jcou.2020.101314.
31. Braccia DJ, Jiang X, Pop M, Hall AB. The capacity to produce hydrogen sulfide (H2S) via cysteine degradation is ubiquitous in the human gut microbiome. Front Microbiol. 2021;12:705583. https://doi.org/10.3389/fmicb.2021.705583.
32. Canyelles M, Borràs C, Rotllan N, et al. Gut microbiota-derived TMAO: a causal factor promoting atherosclerotic cardiovascular disease? Int J Mol Sci. 2023;24:1940. https://doi.org/10.3390/ijms24031940.
33. Wang B, Qiu J, Lian J, et al. Gut metabolite trimethylamine-N-oxide in atherosclerosis: from mechanism to therapy. Front Cardiovasc Med. 2021;8:723886. https://doi.org/10.3389/fcvm.2021.723886.

34. Tennoune N, Andriamihaja M, Blachier F. Production of indole and indole-related compounds by the intestinal microbiota and consequences for the host: the good, the bad, and the ugly. Microorganisms. 2022;10:930. https://doi.org/10.3390/microorganisms10050930.
35. Aldridge DR, Tranah EJ, Shawcross DL. Pathogenesis of hepatic encephalopathy: role of ammonia and systemic inflammation. J Clin Exp Hepatol. 2015;5:S7–S20. https://doi.org/10.1016/j.jceh.2014.06.004.
36. Tang R, Li L. Modulation of short-chain fatty acids as potential therapy method for type 2 diabetes mellitus. Can J Infect Dis Med Microbiol J Can Mal Infect Microbiol Médicale. 2021;2021:6632266. https://doi.org/10.1155/2021/6632266.
37. Guo F-F, Yu T-C, Hong J, Fang J-Y. Emerging roles of hydrogen sulfide in inflammatory and neoplastic colonic diseases. Front Physiol. 2016;7:156. https://doi.org/10.3389/fphys.2016.00156.
38. Beam A, Clinger E, Hao L. Effect of diet and dietary components on the composition of the gut microbiota. Nutrients. 2021;13:2795. https://doi.org/10.3390/nu13082795.
39. Breton J, Galmiche M, Déchelotte P. Dysbiotic gut bacteria in obesity: an overview of the metabolic mechanisms and therapeutic perspectives of next-generation probiotics. Microorganisms. 2022;10:452. https://doi.org/10.3390/microorganisms10020452.
40. Cani PD, Amar J, Iglesias MA, et al. Metabolic endotoxemia initiates obesity and insulin resistance. Diabetes. 2007;56:1761–72. https://doi.org/10.2337/db06-1491.
41. Almeida C, Oliveira R, Soares R, Barata P. Influence of gut microbiota dysbiosis on brain function: a systematic review. Porto Biomed J. 2020;5:1. https://doi.org/10.1097/j.pbj.0000000000000059.
42. Majait S, Nieuwdorp M, Kemper M, Soeters M. The black box orchestra of gut bacteria and bile acids: who is the conductor? Int J Mol Sci. 2023;24:1816. https://doi.org/10.3390/ijms24031816.
43. Vu V, Kim YM, Cho M. Effects of SCFAs and TMAO on non-alcoholic fatty liver disease indicating the therapeutic benefits of plant-based diet, and supplemental prebiotics, probiotics and synbiotics. Appl Biol Chem. 2023;66:11. https://doi.org/10.1186/s13765-022-00755-1.
44. Wu D, Wang H, Xie L, Hu F. Cross-talk between gut microbiota and adipose tissues in obesity and related metabolic diseases. Front Endocrinol. 2022;13:908868. https://doi.org/10.3389/fendo.2022.908868.
45. Kasper P, Martin A, Lang S, et al. NAFLD and cardiovascular diseases: a clinical review. Clin Res Cardiol. 2021;110:921. https://doi.org/10.1007/s00392-020-01709-7.
46. Wang C, Li S, Xue P, et al. The effect of probiotic supplementation on lipid profiles in adults with overweight or obesity: a meta-analysis of randomized controlled trials. J Funct Foods. 2021;86:104711. https://doi.org/10.1016/j.jff.2021.104711.
47. Sun K, Liu Z, Wang H. The effect of probiotics on the serum lipid levels in non-obese healthy adults with hyperlipidemia: a systematic review and meta-analysis of randomized controlled trials. Nutr Hosp. 2022;39:157–70. https://doi.org/10.20960/nh.03688.
48. Pongpirul K, Janchot K, Dai Y. Single strain probiotics for dyslipidemia, fatty liver, and obesity: a systematic review and meta-analysis. World J Meta-Anal. 2019;7:323–38. https://doi.org/10.13105/wjma.v7.i6.323.
49. Karyana IPG, Apsari NLS, Artana IWD, et al. The efficacy of probiotics supplementation on the lipid profiles of obese adolescents: a randomized trial. Bali Med J. 2022;11:540–4. https://doi.org/10.15562/bmj.v11i1.3163.
50. Beserra BTS, Fernandes R, do Rosario VA, et al. A systematic review and meta-analysis of the prebiotics and synbiotics effects on glycaemia, insulin concentrations and lipid parameters in adult patients with overweight or obesity. Clin Nutr. 2015;34:845–58. https://doi.org/10.1016/j.clnu.2014.10.004.
51. Mishima M, Takeda S, Nagane M, et al. Prebiotic effect of poly-D-3-hydroxybutyrate prevents dyslipidemia in obese mice. FASEB J Off Publ Fed Am Soc Exp Biol. 2023;37:e23121. https://doi.org/10.1096/fj.202301191R.
52. Cunningham AL, Stephens JW, Harris DA. Gut microbiota influence in type 2 diabetes mellitus (T2DM). Gut Pathog. 2021;13:1–13. https://doi.org/10.1186/s13099-021-00446-0.

53. Saad MJA, Santos A, Prada PO. Linking gut microbiota and inflammation to obesity and insulin resistance. Physiology. 2016;31:283–93. https://doi.org/10.1152/physiol.00041.2015.
54. Stofan M, Guo GL. Bile acids and FXR: novel targets for liver diseases. Front Med. 2020;7:544.
55. Lun W, Yan Q, Guo X, et al. Mechanism of action of the bile acid receptor TGR5 in obesity. Acta Pharm Sin B. 2023;14:468–91. https://doi.org/10.1016/j.apsb.2023.11.011.
56. Sun L-J, Li J-N, Nie Y-Z. Gut hormones in microbiota-gut-brain cross-talk. Chin Med J. 2020;133:826. https://doi.org/10.1097/CM9.0000000000000706.
57. Salles BIM, Cioffi D, Ferreira SRG. Probiotics supplementation and insulin resistance: a systematic review. Diabetol Metab Syndr. 2020;12:98. https://doi.org/10.1186/s13098-020-00603-6.
58. Zhang Q, Wu Y, Fei X. Effect of probiotics on glucose metabolism in patients with type 2 diabetes mellitus: a meta-analysis of randomized controlled trials. Medicina (Mex). 2016;52:28–34. https://doi.org/10.1016/j.medici.2015.11.008.
59. Li Y, Wu Y, Wu L, et al. The effects of probiotic administration on patients with prediabetes: a meta-analysis and systematic review. J Transl Med. 2022;20:498. https://doi.org/10.1186/s12967-022-03695-y.
60. Pan Y-Q, Zheng Q-X, Jiang X-M, et al. Probiotic supplements improve blood glucose and insulin resistance/sensitivity among healthy and GDM pregnant women: a systematic review and meta-analysis of randomized controlled trials. Evid Based Complement Alternat Med. 2021;2021:e9830200. https://doi.org/10.1155/2021/9830200.
61. Robertson MD. Prebiotics and type 2 diabetes: targeting the gut microbiota for improved glycaemic control? Pract Diabetes. 2020;37:133–7. https://doi.org/10.1002/pdi.2285.
62. Bielka W, Przezak A, Pawlik A. The role of the gut microbiota in the pathogenesis of diabetes. Int J Mol Sci. 2022;23:480. https://doi.org/10.3390/ijms23010480.
63. Morse ZJ, Simister RL, Crowe SA, et al. Virus induced dysbiosis promotes type 1 diabetes onset. Front Immunol. 2023;14:1096323. https://doi.org/10.3389/fimmu.2023.1096323.
64. Zeng Y, Mtintsilana A, Goedecke JH, et al. Alterations in the metabolism of phospholipids, bile acids and branched-chain amino acids predicts development of type 2 diabetes in black south African women: a prospective cohort study. Metabolism. 2019;95:57–64. https://doi.org/10.1016/j.metabol.2019.04.001.
65. Iatcu CO, Steen A, Covasa M. Gut microbiota and complications of type-2 diabetes. Nutrients. 2021;14:166. https://doi.org/10.3390/nu14010166.
66. Li G, Feng H, Mao X-L, et al. The effects of probiotics supplementation on glycaemic control among adults with type 2 diabetes mellitus: a systematic review and meta-analysis of randomised clinical trials. J Transl Med. 2023;21:442. https://doi.org/10.1186/s12967-023-04306-0.
67. Mishra S, Wang S, Nagpal R, et al. Probiotics and prebiotics for the amelioration of type 1 diabetes: present and future perspectives. Microorganisms. 2019;7:67. https://doi.org/10.3390/microorganisms7030067.
68. Kumar S, Kumar R, Rohilla L, et al. A high potency multi-strain probiotic improves glycemic control in children with new-onset type 1 diabetes mellitus: a randomized, double-blind, and placebo-controlled pilot study. Pediatr Diabetes. 2021;22:1014–22. https://doi.org/10.1111/pedi.13244.
69. Ayesha IE, Monson NR, Klair N, et al. Probiotics and their role in the management of type 2 diabetes mellitus (short-term versus long-term effect): a systematic review and meta-analysis. Cureus. 2023;15:e46741. https://doi.org/10.7759/cureus.46741.
70. Pellegrino A, Coppola G, Santopaolo F, et al. Role of Akkermansia in human diseases: from causation to therapeutic properties. Nutrients. 2023;15:1815. https://doi.org/10.3390/nu15081815.
71. Vitetta L, Gorgani NN, Vitetta G, Henson JD. Prebiotics progress shifts in the intestinal microbiome that benefits patients with type 2 diabetes mellitus. Biomol Ther. 2023;13:1307. https://doi.org/10.3390/biom13091307.
72. Tokarek J, Budny E, Saar M, et al. Does the composition of gut microbiota affect hypertension? Molecular mechanisms involved in increasing blood pressure. Int J Mol Sci. 2023;24:1377. https://doi.org/10.3390/ijms24021377.

73. Sun D, Xiang H, Yan J, He L. Intestinal microbiota: a promising therapeutic target for hypertension. Front Cardiovasc Med. 2022;9:970036. https://doi.org/10.3389/fcvm.2022.970036.
74. Elijovich F, Laffer CL, Sahinoz M, et al. The gut microbiome, inflammation, and salt-sensitive hypertension. Curr Hypertens Rep. 2020;22:1–5. https://doi.org/10.1007/s11906-020-01091-9.
75. Verhaar BJH, Prodan A, Nieuwdorp M, Muller M. Gut microbiota in hypertension and atherosclerosis: a review. Nutrients. 2020;12:2982. https://doi.org/10.3390/nu12102982.
76. Apte M, Nadavade N, Sheikh SS. A review on nitrates' health benefits and disease prevention. Nitric Oxide. 2024;142:1–15. https://doi.org/10.1016/j.niox.2023.11.003.
77. Cookson TA. Bacterial-induced blood pressure reduction: mechanisms for the treatment of hypertension via the gut. Front Cardiovasc Med. 2021;8:721393. https://doi.org/10.3389/fcvm.2021.721393.
78. Wang H, Luo Q, Ding X, et al. Trimethylamine N-oxide and its precursors in relation to blood pressure: a mendelian randomization study. Front Cardiovasc Med. 2022;9:922441. https://doi.org/10.3389/fcvm.2022.922441.
79. Zarezadeh M, Musazadeh V, Ghalichi F, et al. Effects of probiotics supplementation on blood pressure: an umbrella meta-analysis of randomized controlled trials. Nutr Metab Cardiovasc Dis. 2023;33:275–86. https://doi.org/10.1016/j.numecd.2022.09.005.
80. Markowiak-Kopeć P, Śliżewska K. The effect of probiotics on the production of short-chain fatty acids by human intestinal microbiome. Nutrients. 2020;12:1107. https://doi.org/10.3390/nu12041107.
81. Liska DJ, Dioum E, Chu Y, Mah E. Narrative review on the effects of oat and sprouted oat components on blood pressure. Nutrients. 2022;14:4772. https://doi.org/10.3390/nu14224772.
82. Honda K, Littman DR. The microbiota in adaptive immune homeostasis and disease. Nature. 2016;535:75–84. https://doi.org/10.1038/nature18848.
83. Lim YJ, Sidor NA, Tonial NC, et al. Uremic toxins in the progression of chronic kidney disease and cardiovascular disease: mechanisms and therapeutic targets. Toxins. 2021;13:142. https://doi.org/10.3390/toxins13020142.
84. Khiabani SA, Asgharzadeh M, Kafil HS. Chronic kidney disease and gut microbiota. Heliyon. 2023;9:e18991. https://doi.org/10.1016/j.heliyon.2023.e18991.
85. Zhao J, Ning X, Liu B, et al. Specific alterations in gut microbiota in patients with chronic kidney disease: an updated systematic review. Ren Fail. 2021;43:102–12. https://doi.org/10.1080/0886022X.2020.1864404.
86. Tang WHW, Wang Z, Kennedy DJ, et al. Gut microbiota-dependent trimethylamine N-oxide (TMAO) pathway contributes to both development of renal insufficiency and mortality risk in chronic kidney disease. Circ Res. 2015;116:448. https://doi.org/10.1161/CIRCRESAHA.116.305360.
87. Rahman MM, Islam F, Or-Rashid MDH, et al. The gut microbiota (microbiome) in cardiovascular disease and its therapeutic regulation. Front Cell Infect Microbiol. 2022;12:903570. https://doi.org/10.3389/fcimb.2022.903570.
88. Tian N, Li L, Ng JK-C, Li PK-T. The potential benefits and controversies of probiotics use in patients at different stages of chronic kidney disease. Nutrients. 2022;14:4044. https://doi.org/10.3390/nu14194044.
89. Favero C, Ortiz A, Sanchez-Niño MD. Probiotics for kidney disease. Clin Kidney J. 2022;15:1981–6. https://doi.org/10.1093/ckj/sfac056.
90. Tuteja S, Ferguson JF. The gut microbiome and response to cardiovascular drugs. Circ Genomic Precis Med. 2019;12:421–9. https://doi.org/10.1161/CIRCGEN.119.002314.
91. Dias AM, Cordeiro G, Estevinho MM, et al. Gut bacterial microbiome composition and statin intake—a systematic review. Pharmacol Res Perspect. 2020;8:e00601. https://doi.org/10.1002/prp2.601.
92. Yoo HH, Kim IS, Yoo D-H, Kim D-H. Effects of orally administered antibiotics on the bioavailability of amlodipine: gut microbiota-mediated drug interaction. J Hypertens. 2016;34:156–62. https://doi.org/10.1097/HJH.0000000000000773.

93. Haiser HJ, Gootenberg DB, Chatman K, et al. Predicting and manipulating cardiac drug inactivation by the human gut bacterium Eggerthella lenta. Science. 2013;341:295–8. https://doi.org/10.1126/science.1235872.
94. Khan TJ, Ahmed YM, Zamzami MA, et al. Atorvastatin treatment modulates the gut microbiota of the hypercholesterolemic patients. Omics J Integr Biol. 2018;22:154–63. https://doi.org/10.1089/omi.2017.0130.
95. Wu D, Tang X, Ding L, et al. Candesartan attenuates hypertension-associated pathophysiological alterations in the gut. Biomed Pharmacother. 2019;116:109040. https://doi.org/10.1016/j.biopha.2019.109040.
96. Kim IS, Yoo D-H, Jung I-H, et al. Reduced metabolic activity of gut microbiota by antibiotics can potentiate the antithrombotic effect of aspirin. Biochem Pharmacol. 2016;122:72–9. https://doi.org/10.1016/j.bcp.2016.09.023.

Microbiota and Gynecological Diseases

8

Sara Morejón-Ruiz and Óscar Martín-Delgado-Sellers

8.1 Introduction

The relationship between gastrointestinal health and various medical conditions has been a topic of growing interest within the medical and scientific community. In this context, one concept that has emerged as a critical factor is "dysbiosis." Dysbiosis refers to an imbalance in the composition and function of the microbiota. While this phenomenon can manifest in various parts of the body, it is closely linked to gastrointestinal health.

This presentation aims to explore the interconnection between dysbiosis and various gynecological diseases and conditions related to women's health. These include polycystic ovary syndrome (PCOS), endometriosis, cervical disorders, alterations in vaginal mucus barrier, and menopause-related conditions. Intestinal dysbiosis and its relationship with these gynecological diseases and disorders have emerged as a key area of research. Recent studies have shed light on how the microbial balance in the gut can influence the development and progression of these conditions, offering an exciting opportunity to better understand these diseases and enhance treatment strategies.

Throughout this presentation, we will delve into the definitions of each disease, their epidemiology, classifications, pathophysiology, hallmark clinical manifestations, and available treatments. Additionally, we will emphasize how intestinal dysbiosis, often underestimated, can play a crucial role in the development and management of these conditions.

S. Morejón-Ruiz (✉)
Department of Surgery, Henares University Hospital, Madrid, Spain
e-mail: sara.morejon@salud.madrid.org

Ó. Martín-Delgado-Sellers
Department of Anesthesiology, Henares University Hospital, Madrid, Spain

Medical Practices, Francisco de Vitoria University, Madrid, Spain
e-mail: oscar.martindelqado@salud.madrid.org

J. Ruiz-Tovar (ed.), *Dysbiosis*, https://doi.org/10.1007/978-3-031-65650-7_8

We hope that this chapter provides a clear insight into intestinal dysbiosis and its impact on women's health while fostering a greater understanding of how microbial imbalances can influence these conditions, paving the way for more effective and personalized treatment approaches.

8.2 Dysbiosis

Definition Dysbiosis is a term used to describe an abnormal imbalance in the composition and function of the microbiota, which is the community of microorganisms, primarily bacteria, inhabiting a biological environment, such as the gastrointestinal tract. Dysbiosis can occur in various parts of the body but is most commonly associated with the intestine.

Epidemiology The epidemiology of dysbiosis is diverse and depends on the location and specific causes of the imbalance. It can affect individuals of all ages, and factors such as diet, antibiotic use, diseases, and other influences contribute to its prevalence.

Classification Dysbiosis can be classified into various types based on its location and causes. Some examples include the following:

- Intestinal dysbiosis: Changes in the gut microbiota.
- Vaginal dysbiosis: Alterations in the vaginal microbiota.
- Oral dysbiosis: Imbalances in the oral microbiota.
- Cutaneous dysbiosis: Changes in the skin microbiota.

Pathophysiology The pathophysiology of dysbiosis involves an alteration in the diversity and balance of bacteria and other microorganisms within a community. It can be related to factors such as diet, antibiotic use, diseases, infections, and changes in the local environment. This imbalance can lead to an increase in harmful microorganisms or a decrease in beneficial bacteria.

Clinical Manifestations Some common symptoms may include the following:

- Gastrointestinal problems, such as bloating, diarrhea, or constipation.
- Recurrent or chronic infections.
- Changes in digestion and nutrient absorption.
- Skin symptoms, such as rashes or acne.
- Changes in vaginal health, such as recurrent yeast or bacterial infections.

Treatment The treatment of dysbiosis depends on the location and underlying cause of the imbalance. It may include the following:

- Dietary changes to promote microbiota health.
- Probiotic supplements to reintroduce beneficial bacteria.
- Treatment of infections or other underlying conditions.
- Lifestyle modifications, such as reducing stress or avoiding excessive antibiotic use.

8.3 Polycystic Ovary Syndrome (PCOS)

Definition Polycystic ovary syndrome (PCOS) is a medical condition that affects women and is characterized by a range of symptoms and findings, including hormonal imbalances and ovarian cysts. It is characterized by a combination of symptoms, including the presence of cysts in the ovaries, irregular menstrual cycles, and hormonal imbalances.

Epidemiology PCOS is one of the most common gynecological conditions in women of reproductive age. It affects approximately 5–10% of women worldwide. The prevalence of polycystic ovary syndrome (PCOS) varies depending on the studied population and the diagnostic criteria used. It is estimated that PCOS affects approximately 5–10% of women of reproductive age worldwide. However, this figure may be higher in certain population groups. It's important to note that PCOS is one of the most common gynecological conditions in women of childbearing age. Prevalence may vary depending on factors such as geographic location, ethnicity, and other demographic factors.

Classification PCOS can be classified into different subtypes based on symptoms and clinical features. These subtypes may include the following:

- PCOS with hyperandrogenism (elevated male hormones).
- PCOS with menstrual irregularities.
- PCOS with insulin resistance.
- Non-hyperandrogenic and non-anovulatory PCOS.

Pathophysiology

The pathophysiology of polycystic ovary syndrome (PCOS) is complex and not yet fully understood, but it involves multiple factors, including the following:

Insulin resistance	Many women with PCOS exhibit insulin resistance, meaning their cells do not respond adequately to insulin, a hormone that regulates blood sugar levels. This insulin resistance can lead to increased insulin production by the pancreas and elevated levels of insulin in the blood
Hyperandrogenism	PCOS is often associated with elevated levels of male hormones, such as testosterone. These hormones can contribute to symptoms such as hirsutism (excessive body hair growth), acne, and hair loss
Hormonal dysregulation	In addition to imbalances in male sex hormones, PCOS also involves changes in female sex hormones like estrogen and progesterone. Hormonal imbalances can affect the menstrual cycle and ovulation
Inflammation	Chronic inflammation has also been implicated in the pathophysiology of PCOS. Systemic inflammation can contribute to insulin resistance and other aspects of the condition
Genetic factors	There is a genetic predisposition to PCOS. Women with a family history of the condition have a higher risk of developing it
Reproductive system	In PCOS, the ovaries often contain multiple small cysts. These are not true cysts but rather immature follicles that do not ovulate correctly. These imbalance in follicle maturation and irregular ovulation are characteristic of PCOS
Environmental factors	Including diet and lifestyle, can also influence the pathophysiology of PCOS. Excess weight, lack of physical activity, and a diet rich in refined carbohydrates can worsen insulin resistance and other aspects of the condition

It's important to note that the pathophysiology of PCOS can vary from one individual to another, making it a complex condition to treat. The management of PCOS often focuses on addressing specific symptoms and underlying factors such as insulin resistance and hormonal imbalances through lifestyle changes, medications, and, in some cases, surgery.

8.4 Clinical Manifestations

Polycystic ovary syndrome (PCOS) can present a wide range of clinical manifestations that vary from one person to another. Some of the most common symptoms and clinical manifestations of PCOS include the following:

Irregular menstrual cycles	Can manifest as absent, infrequent, or very heavy periods
Hirsutism	Excessive facial and body hair growth, especially in areas where men typically have hair, such as the face, chest, back, and abdomen
Acne	Development of acne on the face, chest, and back
Hair loss	Some women with PCOS may experience thinning or loss of hair on the scalp
Weight gain:	Often associated with insulin resistance
Insulin resistance	Increased insulin levels in the blood due to insulin resistance, which can lead to a higher risk of type 2 diabetes

Difficulty getting pregnant	Many women with PCOS have difficulty conceiving due to irregular ovulation
Pelvic pain	Some women may experience pain in the lower abdomen, which may be related to ovarian cysts or inflammation
Mood changes	Such as depression, anxiety, or irritability
Skin issues	Dark skin patches, oily skin, or acanthosis nigricans (a skin condition characterized by dark patches and thickening of the skin)

It is important to note that not all women with PCOS experience all of these symptoms, and the severity of symptoms can vary considerably. Additionally, PCOS not only affects reproductive health but can also have implications for long-term health, such as an increased risk of cardiovascular diseases and type 2 diabetes.

The diagnosis and treatment of polycystic ovary syndrome (PCOS) should be individualized and supervised by a healthcare professional since they may include approaches to address specific symptoms and underlying factors such as insulin resistance and hormonal imbalances.

The treatment of polycystic ovary syndrome (PCOS) focuses on addressing the specific symptoms of each patient and their individual goals, as symptoms can vary widely. Some treatment approaches and options for PCOS include the following:

Lifestyle changes: Weight loss, if necessary, can improve menstrual cycle regulation and reduce insulin resistance, adopting a balanced, low-refined-carbohydrate diet can help regulate insulin levels, and regular exercise can improve insulin sensitivity and contribute to weight loss.

Oral contraceptives: Oral contraceptives (birth control pills) are often prescribed to regulate menstrual cycles and reduce hirsutism and acne symptoms.

Anti-androgens: In cases of hirsutism (excessive hair growth) or severe acne, anti-androgen medications may be prescribed to reduce male hormone levels.

Ovulation-inducing medications: For women looking to get pregnant, medications such as clomiphene citrate or metformin may be used to induce ovulation.

Insulin inhibitors: Metformin, a medication commonly used to treat type 2 diabetes, can help improve insulin sensitivity and regulate menstrual cycles.

Ovarian surgery: In severe cases where other treatments have not been successful, surgery may be performed to remove ovarian cysts or undergo laparoscopic ovarian reduction to improve fertility.

8.5 Endometriosis

Definition Endometriosis is a medical condition in which the tissue that normally lines the inside of the uterus (called the endometrium) grows outside of the uterus. This tissue can be found in other parts of the pelvis, such as the ovaries, fallopian tubes, bladder, or intestines, and it can lead to inflammation, pain, and the formation of scar tissue.

Epidemiology Endometriosis is a common condition in women of reproductive age. It is estimated to affect approximately 10% of women worldwide. It can manifest in women of various ages but is often diagnosed in women between 25 and 35 years of age.

Classification Endometriosis is classified into different stages based on the severity of the disease. The most commonly used classification is the American Society for Reproductive Medicine classification (stages I–IV), which is based on the location, size, and depth of the lesions.

Pathophysiology

The pathophysiology of endometriosis involves the abnormal presence of endometrial tissue outside the uterus. It is believed that endometrial cells travel to other organs through retrograde menstrual flow, where they attach and grow. In addition, genetic, immunological, and hormonal factors also play a role in its development.

Endometriosis is a chronic gynecological disease that can present a variety of clinical manifestations. Symptoms of endometriosis can vary in intensity and severity from one woman to another. Some common clinical manifestations of endometriosis include the following:

Pelvic pain	The most characteristic symptom of endometriosis. This pain is often described as sharp, stabbing, and colicky, and it typically occurs in the lower abdomen and pelvis. Pain may worsen during menstruation and can persist outside of the menstrual period
Dysmenorrhea	Intense menstrual pain and is often associated with endometriosis. Women with endometriosis may experience severe menstrual cramps
Dyspareunia	Pain during or after sexual intercourse
Abnormal bleeding	Which may include bleeding between menstrual periods or heavy menstrual bleeding
Gastrointestinal issues	Endometriosis affecting the intestines or rectum can lead to gastrointestinal symptoms like pain during bowel movements, diarrhea, constipation, or blood in the stool
Infertility	Endometriosis can be a cause of infertility in some women since the condition can affect the fallopian tubes, ovaries, and the uterus, interfering with fertilization and egg implantation
Fatigue	Chronic pain and other endometriosis symptoms can lead to persistent fatigue
Changes in menstrual patterns	Some women with endometriosis may experience changes in the duration and regularity of their menstrual cycles
Urinary symptoms	In rare cases, endometriosis can affect the bladder and result in symptoms such as urinary urgency, pain during urination, or blood in the urine

It's important to note that endometriosis symptoms can vary, and in some cases, the disease can be asymptomatic.

Treatment

The treatment of endometriosis can vary based on the severity of the disease and the specific clinical manifestations experienced by each patient. Below is a summary of treatment options based on the clinical manifestations of endometriosis:

Pelvic pain and dysmenorrhea	Analgesics and oral contraceptives: These may help reduce pain and control the growth of endometrial tissue outside the uterus
Abnormal bleeding	Oral contraceptives or intrauterine devices (IUDs): Regulate bleeding and alleviate symptoms
Changes in menstrual patterns	Oral contraceptives or IUDs
Infertility	Treatment options for infertility related to endometriosis may include controlled ovarian stimulation (COS), intrauterine insemination (IUI), or in vitro fertilization (IVF). The choice of treatment depends on the severity of endometriosis and individual factors
Gastrointestinal issues	If endometriosis affects the intestines, surgery may be necessary to remove affected tissue and make repairs
Urinary symptoms	In severe cases where endometriosis affects the bladder, surgery may be performed to remove the affected tissue

8.6 Cervical Disorders

Cervical disorders can be related to intestinal dysbiosis, although the connection is not always direct.

Recurrent Cervical Infections

- **Clinical Presentation:** Recurrent cervical infections may manifest with symptoms such as abnormal vaginal discharge, pelvic pain, changes in menstrual bleeding, and discomfort during sexual intercourse. These infections can be caused by various pathogens, such as the human papillomavirus (HPV), bacteria, or fungi.
- **Incidence:** The incidence of recurrent cervical infections varies depending on the population and individual risk factors. Rates are higher in sexually active women.
- **Treatment:** Treatment depends on the underlying cause. For example, bacterial infections may require antibiotics, while fungal infections can be treated with

antifungals. Prevention through safe sexual practices and HPV vaccination is an important measure.

Cervical Dysplasia

- **Clinical Presentation:** Cervical dysplasia is a term used to describe abnormal cellular changes in the cervix. It may not present symptoms, but in advanced stages, it can lead to abnormal bleeding, pelvic pain, and, in severe cases, cervical cancer.
- **Incidence:** The incidence of cervical dysplasia varies but is associated with persistent HPV infection and other risk factors. HPV is a common sexually transmitted infection.
- **Treatment:** Treatment of cervical dysplasia depends on the severity of the lesions. It may include procedures like electrocautery excision or laser ablation. Early detection and follow-up are key to cervical cancer prevention.

The relationship between intestinal dysbiosis and cervical pathology is complex and generally indirect, as imbalances in intestinal microbiota can influence immunity and a person's overall health. Treatment focuses on addressing the specific conditions affecting cervical health and may include antimicrobial therapy, dietary and lifestyle changes, and preventive measures such as HPV vaccination.

8.7 Cervical Mucus Alterations

Definition Cervical mucus alterations are abnormal changes in the characteristics of cervical mucus, which is the secretion produced by the cervix throughout the menstrual cycle. These changes can affect a woman's fertility and gynecological health.

Epidemiological Factors

1. **Individual Risk Factors**: The incidence and prevalence of cervical mucus alterations related to intestinal dysbiosis can be influenced by factors such as age, hormonal status, overall health, and an individual's medical history. For example, women of childbearing age may experience changes in cervical mucus related to menstrual cycles and hormonal imbalances.
2. **Vaginal Infections**: Vaginal infections such as bacterial vaginosis and yeast infections can alter the composition and quality of cervical mucus. The incidence of these infections may vary depending on the population and individual risk factors. Recurrent vaginal infections can contribute to changes in cervical mucus.

3. **Diet and Lifestyle**: A person's diet and lifestyle can also influence intestinal microbiota and, ultimately, cervical mucus. For example, a diet rich in fiber and low in saturated fats can promote a healthy balance in intestinal microbiota, which can have a positive impact on cervical health.
4. **Antibiotic Use**: Excessive or inappropriate use of antibiotics can alter intestinal microbiota and increase the risk of vaginal infections and changes in cervical mucus. This may be more relevant in populations that tend to use antibiotics frequently.
5. **Geographic and Social Factors**: The incidence of cervical mucus alterations related to dysbiosis may vary geographically and be influenced by socioeconomic and cultural factors. For example, rates of vaginal infections may be higher in areas with limited access to healthcare and sexual health education.

It's important to note that these alterations can manifest in different ways and may not necessarily be a specific diagnosis but rather a symptom or finding during gynecological evaluation. The precise relationship between intestinal dysbiosis and cervical mucus alterations is being further investigated and understood, and epidemiology may vary based on new scientific discoveries and clinical findings.

Classification Cervical mucus alterations can be classified into different categories based on their specific characteristics. Some examples include scant or insufficient cervical mucus, thick or viscous cervical mucus, and changes in the consistency of cervical mucus throughout the menstrual cycle.

Pathophysiology The pathophysiology of cervical mucus alterations may be related to hormonal factors, infections, inflammation, or underlying medical conditions. For instance, taking certain medications such as oral contraceptives can affect the production and quality of cervical mucus.

Clinical Manifestations Clinical manifestations of cervical mucus alterations can vary depending on the type of change in cervical mucus. Some symptoms or signs may include the following:

- Vaginal dryness
- Difficulty conceiving due to thick cervical mucus that hinders sperm passage
- Changes in the quality and quantity of cervical mucus throughout the menstrual cycle.

Cervical mucus alterations related to dysbiosis can manifest in various ways and may be linked to a variety of factors. Here are some types of cervical mucus alterations and their possible treatments based on pathophysiology:

- Treatment: Treatment may include correcting intestinal dysbiosis through dietary changes, incorporating probiotics that promote a healthy balance in microbiota, and eliminating factors contributing to dysbiosis, such as overuse of antibiotics.

8.8 Menopause

Menopause and its relationship with dysbiosis are associated with hormonal and microbiological changes in women's bodies.

Definition Menopause is a natural stage in a woman's life that marks the permanent cessation of menstruation and a decrease in the production of hormones such as estrogen and progesterone.

Epidemiology Menopause generally occurs in women between the ages of 45 and 55, although the age can vary. Dysbiosis in the intestine is a phenomenon that can affect people of all ages but may become more common with age.

Classification Menopause is classified into different stages, including perimenopause (the transitional stage before menopause) and postmenopause (after menopause).

Pathophysiology The relationship between menopause and intestinal dysbiosis involves a series of factors that affect the composition and function of intestinal microbiota in postmenopausal women. The pathophysiology of this relationship can be explained as follows:

1. Hormonal Changes: During menopause, there is a significant decrease in the production of sex hormones like estrogen and progesterone. These hormones play a crucial role in regulating various systems in the body, including the immune system and the balance of intestinal microbiota.
2. Impact on the Immune System: Hormonal changes associated with menopause can affect the immune system of women. This can lead to an altered immune response in the gut, which can, in turn, influence the composition of microbiota.
3. Chronic Inflammation: Menopause is associated with a higher risk of low-grade chronic inflammation that can negatively affect intestinal health and microbiota diversity.
4. Medication Use: During menopause, it is common for women to receive treatment with hormone replacement therapy or other medications. Some of these medications can influence intestinal microbiota.
5. Impact on the Intestinal Barrier: Intestinal microbiota plays a role in maintaining the intestinal barrier, which protects the gut from harmful substances. Changes

in microbiota can weaken this barrier, leading to an increased risk of intestinal permeability and the passage of bacteria and bacterial products into the bloodstream.

6. Association with Age-Related Diseases: Menopause is associated with a higher risk of age-related chronic diseases such as osteoporosis and cardiovascular diseases. These diseases can influence intestinal health and microbiota composition.

In summary, menopause can lead to hormonal, immunological, inflammatory, dietary, and lifestyle changes that affect intestinal microbiota. Intestinal dysbiosis in postmenopausal women can contribute to a range of health issues, such as gastrointestinal disorders and a higher risk of chronic diseases. Treating intestinal dysbiosis in this context may involve dietary changes, probiotic supplements, and lifestyle modifications to promote a healthy and balanced intestinal microbiota.

The treatment of menopause in relation to intestinal dysbiosis focuses on alleviating menopausal symptoms while addressing intestinal microbiota balance. Here are some considerations:

Hormone replacement therapy (HRT)	Is a common approach to alleviate menopausal symptoms like hot flashes and vaginal dryness. However, the use of HRT can have effects on intestinal microbiota
Dietary modification	Adopting a balanced diet rich in fiber, fruits, vegetables, and fermented foods can be beneficial for intestinal health during menopause
Probiotic and prebiotic supplements	Can help maintain a healthy balance of intestinal microbiota. Probiotics can help reintroduce beneficial bacteria, while prebiotics are foods that encourage their growth
Stress management	Chronic stress can negatively impact intestinal health. Meditation, yoga, and other stress management techniques can be helpful
Avoid excessive alcohol and tobacco use	Alcohol and tobacco can have adverse effects on intestinal health

In summary, the treatment of menopause in relation to intestinal dysbiosis involves addressing both menopausal symptoms and intestinal microbiota balance. A combination of dietary approaches, a healthy lifestyle, and, in some cases, probiotic supplements can contribute to a more balanced intestinal microbiota during this life stage.

8.9 Vaginal Bacteriosis

Bacterial vaginosis (BV) is a common vaginal infection characterized by an imbalance in vaginal microbiota, where beneficial bacteria are reduced and harmful bacteria increase. Although it's a vaginal condition, its relationship with intestinal dysbiosis is relevant.

Intestinal dysbiosis can indirectly affect vaginal microbiota by triggering systemic changes in the body. An imbalance in intestinal microbiota can weaken the immune system and increase susceptibility to infections, including bacterial vaginosis.

Research is ongoing to better understand this relationship, but it's important to recognize that intestinal and vaginal health are often interconnected, and balance in both areas is essential for overall gynecological health.

The treatment for bacterial vaginosis often involves the use of specific antibiotics and restoring the balance of vaginal microbiota through probiotics and prebiotics.

Treatment for bacterial vaginosis (BV) in relation to intestinal dysbiosis can involve a comprehensive approach that addresses both vaginal balance and intestinal microbiota. Here are some considerations:

Treatment of bacterial vaginosis (BV)	The primary treatment for BV usually involves the prescription of oral antibiotics or vaginal gel with antibiotics, such as metronidazole or clindamycin. These medications help eliminate unwanted bacteria in the vagina
Vaginal probiotics	Vaginal probiotics are being investigated as a promising approach to help restore the balance of vaginal microbiota. These products contain strains of beneficial bacteria that can help prevent the recurrence of BV
Diet modification	Since there is a connection between intestinal and vaginal microbiota, maintaining a balanced diet that promotes intestinal health can also be beneficial for preventing BV. A diet rich in fiber and prebiotic foods can help maintain a healthy gut
Probiotic supplements	Taking oral probiotics containing beneficial strains like *lactobacillus* can contribute to the balance of intestinal microbiota and, by extension, vaginal microbiota
Adequate vaginal hygiene	Using appropriate hygiene products and avoiding the use of vaginal douches, which can disrupt the natural balance of the vagina, is important for preventing BV

8.10 Conclusion

The interconnection between intestinal dysbiosis and gynecological diseases, including vaginosis, is an important area of research in medicine. Dysbiosis can influence the onset and severity of these conditions. Understanding the pathophysiology and microbiota is crucial for improving diagnosis and treatment. A multidisciplinary approach that addresses both intestinal and gynecological health is essential to provide comprehensive and personalized treatment for patients. Future research will shed light on the complex relationship between microbiota and gynecological health, providing opportunities to improve the quality of life for women.

Suggested Readings

1. Schlienger J-L. Disbiosis intestinal y enfermedades metabólicas. Capítulo 14. In: Diabetología. 3rd ed. España: Elsevier; 2023. p. 353–9. Disponible en: https://www-clinicalkey-es.bvcscm.a17.csinet.es/#!/content/book/3-s2.0-B9788491136750000140?scrollTo=%23hl0000101.
2. Sobstyl A, Chałupnik A, Mertowska P, Grywalska E. How do microorganisms influence the development of endometriosis? participation of genital, intestinal and oral microbiota in metabolic regulation and immunopathogenesis of endometriosis. Int J Mol Sci. 2023;24:10920. Clinicalkey.es. [citado el 19 de octubre de 2023]. Disponible en: https://www.clinicalkey.es/#!/content/medline/2-s2.0-37446108
3. Lingaiah S, Arffman RK, Morin-Papunen L, Tapanainen JS, Piltonen T. Markers of gastrointestinal permeability and dysbiosis in premenopausal women with PCOS: a case-control study. BMJ Open. 2021;11:e045324. Disponible en: https://www-clinicalkey-es.bvcscm.a17.csinet.es/#!/content/medline/2-s2.0-34226215
4. Wahid M, Dar SA, Jawed A, Mandal RK, Akhter N, Khan S, Khan F, Jogaiah S, Rai AK, Rattan R. Microbes in gynecologic cancers: causes or consequences and therapeutic potential. In: Seminars in cancer biology 86. Amsterdam: Elsevier; 2021. [citado el 19 de octubre de 2023]. Disponible en: https://www.clinicalkey.es/#!/content/journal/1-s2.0-S1044579X2100208X.
5. Chu J, Feng S, Guo C, Xue B, He K, Li L. Immunological mechanisms of inflammatory diseases caused by gut microbiota dysbiosis: a review. Biomed Pharmacother. 2023;164:114985. Disponible en: https://www-clinicalkey-es.bvcscm.a17.csinet.es/#!/content/journal/1-s2.0-S0753332223007758

9 Microbiota and Cancer

Ines Macias-Gamero

9.1 Introduction to Cancer and the Microbiota

Cancer is a broad term to describe a group of diseases characterized by uncontrolled proliferation of abnormal cells within the body, leading to the formation of malignant tumors or the infiltration of cancerous cells into normal tissues [1]. Cancer can occur virtually in any tissue or organ in the body. Understanding the causes and progression of cancer is paramount in the field of oncology, as it not only aids in early detection and effective treatment but also offers opportunities for prevention and improved patient outcomes [2].

Cancer accounts for a substantial portion of the global disease burden, causing significant morbidity and mortality worldwide [3]. Moreover, the economic and social costs associated with cancer care and its consequences are substantial, underscoring the urgency of advancing our knowledge in this field [4].

In recent years, research has unveiled a fascinating aspect of cancer development and progression—the intricate relationship between the human microbiota and cancer. The microbiota, which refers to the diverse community of microorganisms residing in and on the human body, has emerged as a critical player in the maintenance of health and the pathogenesis of various diseases, including cancer [5].

The human microbiota comprises a vast array of bacteria, viruses, fungi, and other microorganisms that colonize different anatomical sites, such as the gut, skin, oral cavity, and more [6]. It exerts a profound influence on host physiology and immune function, participating in processes such as digestion, nutrient metabolism, and immune system modulation [7].

Consequently, disruptions in the delicate balance of the microbiota can have far-reaching implications for human health, including increased susceptibility to various diseases [8]. Research in this field has illuminated how alterations in the

I. Macias-Gamero (✉)
Department of Biomedicine, Universidad Alfonso X El Sabio, Madrid, Spain

J. Ruiz-Tovar (ed.), *Dysbiosis*, https://doi.org/10.1007/978-3-031-65650-7_9

microbiota composition and function can influence cancer risk, tumor development, and responses to cancer therapy [9]. This interplay between the microbiota and cancer has opened up new avenues for preventive strategies, therapeutic interventions, and personalized medicine approaches [10].

In this chapter, we will delve deeper into the intricate relationship between cancer and the microbiota, exploring the mechanisms underlying their interactions, their impact on cancer risk and progression, and the potential implications for cancer prevention and treatment.

9.2 Microbiota Composition

The human microbiota is a diverse and dynamic community of microorganisms that inhabits various body sites. This microbial consortium comprises a wide array of bacteria, viruses, fungi, archaea, and other microorganisms that coexist with the human host. Its composition varies across different anatomical locations, reflecting the specific environmental conditions and functional requirements of each site [11].

One of the most extensively studied components of the human microbiota is the gut microbiota. The human gastrointestinal tract houses trillions of microorganisms, primarily bacteria, which assist in digestion, nutrient absorption, and the synthesis of various metabolites [5]. The gut microbiota is highly complex and composed of several dominant bacterial phyla, including *Firmicutes*, *Bacteroidetes*, *Proteobacteria*, and *Actinobacteria*. Each of these phyla comprises numerous genera and species, contributing to the overall diversity of the gut microbiota [12].

Apart from the gut, the human microbiota is present in other sites. The skin, the body's largest organ, harbors a diverse microbiota consisting of bacteria, fungi, and viruses. *Staphylococcus*, *Propionibacterium*, and *Corynebacterium* are some of the prominent bacterial genera inhabiting the skin [13]. In the oral cavity, microbial communities are vital for maintaining oral health and contribute to processes like digestion. Bacterial species like *Streptococcus*, *Actinomyces*, and *Prevotella* are common oral inhabitants [14].

Advancements in sequencing technologies have revolutionized our understanding of microbiota composition. High-throughput sequencing methods, such as 16S rRNA gene sequencing and metagenomic sequencing, have allowed for the comprehensive analysis of microbial communities. 16S rRNA gene sequencing targets a conserved region in bacterial genomes, enabling the identification of different bacterial taxa [15]. Metagenomic sequencing, on the other hand, provides a broader view of microbial communities by sequencing all genetic material present, allowing the characterization of not only bacteria but also viruses, fungi, and archaea [16]. These techniques have provided insights into the rich diversity and functional potential of the human microbiota across various body sites.

Understanding microbiota composition and its variations among individuals and populations is crucial in unraveling its role in health and disease. It sets the stage for investigating how alterations in microbiota composition may influence susceptibility to various conditions, including cancer, and provides the basis for developing strategies to modulate the microbiota for therapeutic purposes.

9.3 Microbiota-Gut-Immune System Axis

The microbiota-gut-immune system axis is a critical and dynamic interface within the human body that orchestrates a complex and mutually beneficial relationship between the gut microbiota and the immune system. This axis plays a pivotal role in influencing overall health, immune function, and maintaining homeostasis. Understanding this intricate interplay is fundamental to appreciating the profound impact of the gut microbiota on human well-being [7].

9.3.1 Interaction Between Gut Microbiota and the Immune System

The gut microbiota interacts with the immune system in several ways. One of the primary mechanisms is through the recognition of microbe-associated molecular patterns (MAMPs) by pattern recognition receptors (PRRs) on immune cells. The presence of beneficial gut bacteria helps educate the immune system and fine-tunes its responses, promoting tolerance to harmless microbes and enhancing immunity against pathogens [17].

Moreover, the gut microbiota influences the development and maturation of immune cells in the gut-associated lymphoid tissue (GALT), as well as in distant lymphoid organs. This interaction fosters a balanced immune response and helps prevent aberrant immune reactions, such as allergies or autoimmune diseases [18].

9.3.2 Role of Gut-Associated Lymphoid Tissue (GALT) and Mucosal Immunity

The gut-associated lymphoid tissue (GALT) is a critical component of the microbiota-gut-immune system axis. It encompasses a network of lymphoid structures within the gastrointestinal tract, including Peyer's patches, mesenteric lymph nodes, and isolated lymphoid follicles. GALT serves as the front line of defense against pathogenic microbes and plays a key role in maintaining gut homeostasis [19].

Mucosal immunity, primarily orchestrated by GALT, is designed to protect the mucous membranes of the gut, where the majority of the body's interactions with the external environment occur. This immune system component is finely tuned to distinguish between harmless commensal bacteria and harmful pathogens. Dysregulation of this balance can lead to chronic inflammation and contribute to the development of various diseases, including inflammatory bowel disease (IBD) [20].

Through secretory IgA (sIgA) antibodies, immune cells in GALT actively regulate the composition of the gut microbiota by coating and neutralizing potentially harmful bacteria while allowing commensal microbes to thrive. This complex interaction helps maintain a balanced, diverse microbiota and prevents pathogen overgrowth [20].

9.4 Microbiota and Cancer Risk

Growing evidence suggests a significant link between alterations in the human microbiota and an increased risk of cancer development. This connection has been extensively studied in the context of colorectal cancer, as well as other cancer types, shedding light on the multifaceted mechanisms through which the microbiota may influence cancer risk [9].

9.4.1 Colorectal Cancer and Microbiota

Colorectal cancer, in particular, has been a focus of research regarding the microbiota-cancer connection. Numerous studies have shown that dysbiosis, an imbalance or disruption in the gut microbiota composition, is associated with an elevated risk of colorectal cancer [21]. Specific bacterial species, such as *Fusobacterium nucleatum* and certain strains of *Escherichia coli*, have been implicated in colorectal cancer pathogenesis [22]. Changes in the gut microbiota composition can contribute to chronic inflammation in the colon, which is a well-established risk factor for colorectal cancer [23].

9.4.2 Mechanisms of Microbiota Influence on Cancer Risk

Several mechanisms through which the microbiota can influence cancer risk have been proposed, including the following:

1. **Inflammation**: Chronic inflammation, often triggered by an imbalanced gut microbiota, can promote the development and progression of cancer. Inflammatory responses may induce DNA damage and support the survival of cancer cells, creating a favorable microenvironment for tumor growth [24].
2. **Microbial Metabolites**: The microbiota plays a crucial role in metabolizing dietary components, producing a variety of microbial metabolites. Some of these metabolites, such as short-chain fatty acids (SCFAs), have anti-inflammatory and protective effects against cancer. In contrast, other metabolites, like secondary bile acids, can be pro-carcinogenic and increase cancer risk [25].
3. **Gut Barrier Function**: The gut barrier, which separates the intestinal microbiota from the host's internal tissues, is maintained by a delicate balance of microbial and host factors. Dysbiosis can disrupt this barrier, leading to increased

permeability and the translocation of microbial products, like lipopolysaccharides (LPS), into systemic circulation. This can trigger inflammation and promote cancer development [26].

The microbiota's role in modulating cancer risk extends beyond the gut, as it has been implicated in various cancer types, including hepatocellular carcinoma, pancreatic cancer, and even extraintestinal cancers. While the specific mechanisms may vary, common themes include immune system modulation, inflammation, and the production of microbial metabolites [27].

9.4.3 Hepatocellular Carcinoma (HCC)

Hepatocellular carcinoma is the most common form of liver cancer, and it has been associated with alterations in the gut microbiota. Recent research has shown that the gut microbiota can influence the risk and progression of HCC. Dysbiosis, characterized by changes in microbial diversity and composition, has been observed in patients with HCC. Specifically, the presence of pathogenic bacteria, such as *Escherichia coli* and *Enterococcus faecalis*, has been linked to chronic liver inflammation and fibrosis, which are risk factors for the development of HCC [28].

9.4.4 Pancreatic Cancer

Pancreatic cancer, one of the deadliest forms of cancer, has also shown connections to the gut microbiota. Studies have indicated alterations in the gut microbiota composition in individuals with pancreatic cancer. Dysbiosis in pancreatic cancer often involves a reduction in microbial diversity and an increase in certain bacterial species, such as *Gammaproteobacteria*. The mechanisms through which the gut microbiota influences pancreatic cancer risk are still being explored, but they likely involve inflammation, immune modulation, and the production of microbial metabolites [29].

9.4.5 Gastric Cancer

Helicobacter pylori infection is a well-known risk factor for gastric cancer. However, emerging research suggests that the gut microbiota's composition may also contribute to gastric cancer development. Dysbiosis in gastric cancer often involves an increase in certain bacteria, such as *Fusobacterium* and *Streptococcus* species, which can influence the inflammatory response in the stomach. This chronic inflammation may contribute to gastric cancer risk [30].

9.5 Role of Gut Microbiota in Colorectal Cancer

Colorectal cancer (CRC) is one of the most extensively studied cancer types in the context of the gut microbiota. Research in recent years has revealed a compelling link between the composition of the gut microbiota and the risk of CRC. This relationship is complex and multifaceted, involving specific bacterial species or groups that can either increase or decrease the risk of colorectal cancer [21].

9.5.1 Gut Microbiota Dysbiosis in Colorectal Cancer

Gut microbiota dysbiosis, characterized by an imbalance in the composition and function of the gut microbiota, is a hallmark of CRC. Dysbiosis in the context of CRC often involves a reduction in microbial diversity and alterations in the relative abundance of specific bacterial taxa. One of the consistent observations is an increase in pro-inflammatory bacteria, such as *Fusobacterium nucleatum*, *Escherichia coli*, and certain strains of *Bacteroides fragilis*. These bacteria are associated with chronic inflammation in the gut, which can contribute to the initiation and progression of CRC [22].

9.5.2 Protective Bacterial Species and CRC Risk

Conversely, some bacterial species or groups have shown protective effects against CRC. For example, various strains of *Bifidobacterium* and *Lactobacillus* have been associated with a reduced risk of CRC. These probiotic bacteria can produce short-chain fatty acids (SCFAs), such as butyrate, which have anti-inflammatory and anti-tumor properties and help maintain the health of the colonic mucosa [25].

9.5.3 Mechanisms Underlying the Gut Microbiota-CRC Relationship

The gut microbiota influences CRC risk through several mechanisms, including the following:

1. **Inflammation**: Pro-inflammatory bacteria can trigger inflammation in the colon, promoting the proliferation of cancer cells and the formation of pre-cancerous lesions. Inflammation can also lead to DNA damage and genetic mutations that contribute to CRC development [23].
2. **Microbial Metabolites**: The gut microbiota produces metabolites, such as secondary bile acids and SCFAs, which can influence CRC risk. Secondary bile acids, formed by certain bacteria, can be pro-carcinogenic, while SCFAs have protective effects. They regulate immune responses and maintain the health of the intestinal mucosa [29].

3. **Immune System Modulation**: The gut microbiota interacts with the host immune system, influencing immune responses in the gut. Dysbiosis can lead to immune dysfunction and reduced surveillance against cancerous cells, contributing to CRC development [7].

9.6 Microbiota and Cancer Treatment

The influence of the human microbiota on cancer treatment, including chemotherapy, immunotherapy, and radiation therapy, has garnered significant attention in recent years. Growing evidence suggests that the composition and function of the gut microbiota can impact the efficacy of cancer treatments and influence the severity of treatment-related side effects, thereby offering promising avenues for optimizing cancer therapies [10].

9.6.1 Implications for Chemotherapy

Chemotherapy is a common cancer treatment that often involves the administration of potent drugs. The gut microbiota can influence chemotherapy outcomes through various mechanisms. Some bacteria can metabolize chemotherapy drugs, potentially reducing their effectiveness, while others may promote drug absorption and enhance treatment responses [31].

For example, specific gut bacteria can activate the prodrug irinotecan into its active form but can also inactivate it into an inactive metabolite. The balance of these microbial activities can affect the efficacy of irinotecan-based chemotherapy [32].

9.6.2 Implications for Immunotherapy

Immunotherapy has emerged as a revolutionary approach to cancer treatment, harnessing the immune system to target and destroy cancer cells. The gut microbiota plays a crucial role in modulating the immune system, and research has revealed that certain microbial species can enhance the response to immunotherapy. For instance, some bacteria stimulate the immune system, increasing the effectiveness of immune checkpoint inhibitors, a class of immunotherapy drugs [33].

Furthermore, the gut microbiota can influence the severity of immune-related adverse events associated with immunotherapy. Dysbiosis may exacerbate side effects, while a healthy and diverse gut microbiota might help mitigate these complications [34].

9.6.3 Implications for Radiation Therapy

Radiation therapy uses high-energy rays to target and destroy cancer cells. The gut microbiota's role in radiation therapy is twofold. First, the gut microbiota can influence the response of normal tissues to radiation. Microbial metabolites, such as short-chain fatty acids, can protect healthy tissues from radiation-induced damage. Second, the gut microbiota can modulate systemic immune responses that affect the body's overall response to radiation therapy [35].

9.6.4 Treatment Efficacy and Side Effects

The impact of the gut microbiota on cancer treatment efficacy and side effects underscores the need for a personalized approach to cancer therapy. Manipulating the gut microbiota, through strategies such as probiotics, prebiotics, or fecal microbiota transplantation (FMT), is an area of active investigation. Such interventions aim to enhance treatment outcomes, reduce side effects, and improve patients' quality of life during cancer treatment [36].

9.7 Microbiota Modulation for Cancer Prevention and Therapy

Modulating the gut microbiota has emerged as a promising avenue for both cancer prevention and therapy. The composition and function of the microbiota can significantly impact cancer risk and influence treatment outcomes. Several strategies, including probiotics, prebiotics, dietary interventions, and fecal microbiota transplantation (FMT), offer potential tools for optimizing cancer prevention and therapy [37].

9.7.1 Probiotics

Probiotics are live microorganisms that, when administered in adequate amounts, confer health benefits to the host. Probiotics are being investigated for their potential to prevent cancer by promoting a balanced and beneficial gut microbiota composition. They can also help mitigate some of the gastrointestinal side effects of cancer therapies like chemotherapy and radiation. Specific strains of probiotics have shown promise in modulating inflammation and supporting immune function, which can be beneficial in cancer prevention and during treatment [38].

9.7.2 Prebiotics

Prebiotics are dietary compounds that selectively promote the growth and activity of beneficial gut bacteria. They serve as substrates for beneficial bacteria to produce metabolites like short-chain fatty acids (SCFAs), which have anti-inflammatory and anti-tumor properties. A diet rich in prebiotics, such as fiber from whole grains, vegetables, and fruits, can help maintain a healthy gut microbiota and may reduce the risk of colorectal cancer [39].

9.7.3 Dietary Interventions

Dietary interventions can have a profound impact on the gut microbiota. For example, a diet rich in plant-based foods can promote the growth of beneficial bacteria. On the other hand, diets high in saturated fats, red meat, and processed foods can favor the growth of potentially harmful bacteria associated with cancer risk. Adopting a diet that supports a diverse and balanced gut microbiota can be a valuable strategy for cancer prevention [40].

9.7.4 Fecal Microbiota Transplantation (FMT)

FMT is a more advanced approach involving the transfer of fecal material from a healthy donor to a patient's gastrointestinal tract. FMT has shown promise in the treatment of conditions like *Clostridium difficile* infection, and its potential application in cancer therapy is an area of ongoing research. By introducing a healthy and diverse microbiota, FMT may help restore microbial balance in patients undergoing cancer treatment, potentially improving treatment efficacy and reducing side effects [41].

9.7.5 Modifying Gut Microbiota Dysbiosis in Precision Cancer Treatment

Precision medicine has revolutionized cancer care by tailoring treatments to individual patients based on their unique genetic, molecular, and clinical characteristics. In recent years, an emerging area of interest within precision oncology is the modulation of gut microbiota dysbiosis to enhance the efficacy of cancer treatments. The gut microbiota has been recognized as a dynamic player in cancer, and harnessing its potential offers novel strategies for personalized cancer therapy [1].

9.7.6 Microbial Signatures in Precision Medicine

In the context of precision medicine, researchers are exploring the concept of "microbial signatures." These signatures consist of unique gut microbiota compositions associated with different cancer types, stages, and responses to treatment. The identification of such microbial profiles may help in predicting patient responses to specific cancer therapies. By analyzing the gut microbiota of individual patients, clinicians can gain insights into how to tailor treatments to maximize their effectiveness [2].

9.7.7 Personalized Treatment Approaches

The gut microbiota's role in modulating drug metabolism, immune responses, and inflammation has significant implications for treatment individualization. For example, in immunotherapy, certain microbial profiles are associated with a more favorable response. Thus, strategies to promote or restore these specific microbiota compositions can be part of a personalized treatment plan. Precision medicine allows for the identification of patients who may benefit from microbiota-based interventions, such as probiotics, prebiotics, or fecal microbiota transplantation (FMT), to optimize cancer therapy outcomes [3].

9.7.8 Combination Therapies

In the field of precision oncology, combination therapies are increasingly explored to address the heterogeneity of cancer. Combining traditional treatments with microbiota-based interventions is a promising strategy. For instance, certain bacterial species can influence the metabolism of chemotherapy drugs, and the gut microbiota can modulate immune checkpoint inhibitors' efficacy. Combining microbiota modulation with conventional treatments may enhance overall treatment responses and reduce side effects in a personalized manner [4].

9.7.9 Challenges and Considerations

Despite the exciting potential, precision medicine involving the gut microbiota faces several challenges. Microbiota-based therapies are still in their early stages and require rigorous clinical testing. Moreover, ethical, regulatory, and safety aspects must be addressed. Standardizing protocols for FMT and targeted probiotics, ensuring the safety of microbial materials, and developing guidelines for clinical practice are essential steps [5].

In summary, the integration of gut microbiota modulation within the framework of precision medicine represents a promising frontier in cancer treatment. The microbial signatures of individual patients may guide treatment decisions, leading to more effective, personalized therapies. While challenges exist, this emerging field holds substantial potential for enhancing cancer care through a deeper understanding of the gut microbiota's role in cancer and treatment responses.

9.8 Emerging Research and Future Directions

Recent Research Findings Recent research in the field of cancer and microbiota has uncovered a multitude of intriguing findings. Investigations have revealed the critical role of the gut microbiota in influencing cancer risk, progression, and treatment outcomes. For example, ongoing studies have provided insights into the specific bacterial species associated with various cancer types, such as colorectal cancer and hepatocellular carcinoma, and their impact on disease development. Furthermore, research has elucidated the complex mechanisms by which the microbiota modulates the immune response to cancer and influences the efficacy of immunotherapy. The gut microbiota's role in the metabolism of chemotherapy drugs and its influence on the gut-brain axis are also areas of active exploration [10, 32, 42].

Future Directions The future of research in cancer and microbiota holds great promise. Ongoing studies aim to refine our understanding of the microbiota's role in cancer and identify biomarkers for cancer risk assessment and treatment response prediction. Prospective research also focuses on elucidating the dynamic interplay between the microbiota and various cancer therapies, such as chemotherapy, immunotherapy, and radiation therapy. This knowledge may lead to the development of personalized interventions that optimize treatment outcomes. Moreover, the potential for microbiota modulation, through strategies like FMT and targeted probiotics, represents an exciting avenue for improving cancer care. Future research will need to consider individualized approaches that account for the unique microbial signatures of patients and their specific cancer types, as well as ethical and regulatory aspects that govern microbiota-based interventions [27, 43].

9.9 Clinical Implications and Challenges

Challenges in Translation Translating microbiota research into clinical practice presents several challenges. While the evidence linking microbiota to cancer is compelling, the microbiota is highly dynamic and can vary significantly among individuals. Identifying consistent microbial markers for diagnosis and prognosis remains a challenge. Additionally, large-scale clinical trials are needed to establish the safety and efficacy of microbiota-based interventions, which require significant resources and time. Furthermore, standardizing protocols for FMT and targeted probiotics is crucial, as microbial composition can be influenced by donor variability and preparation methods.

Ethical and Regulatory Aspects The clinical application of microbiota-based therapies raises ethical and regulatory considerations. The safety and long-term consequences of FMT and targeted probiotics require careful assessment, and their potential impact on healthy gut microbiota should be considered. Regulations surrounding the sourcing and processing of microbial materials, such as fecal samples, must be developed and enforced. Additionally, ensuring equitable access to microbiota-based therapies and addressing potential commercialization issues will be essential to prevent disparities in cancer care.

9.10 Conclusion: The Interplay between Cancer and the Gut Microbiota

The interrelationship between cancer and the gut microbiota is a captivating area of study with significant implications for cancer prevention and treatment. The gut microbiota, a diverse collection of microorganisms residing within and on the human body, profoundly influences various physiological processes and plays a crucial role in cancer biology.

9.10.1 Understanding the Complexity of Cancer

Cancer is a complex disease characterized by uncontrolled cell growth, genetic mutations, and intricate molecular interactions. It results from a combination of genetic and environmental factors, and the gut microbiota is a prominent environmental contributor that interacts with the host's genetics to influence cancer risk.

9.10.2 Diverse and Dynamic Microbiota Composition

The human microbiota consists of diverse ecosystems in various body sites, with the gut microbiota being a key player. Advances in sequencing technologies have allowed researchers to identify microbial compositions and their impact on human health and disease. Dysbiosis, characterized by imbalances in microbial communities, is associated with various cancers, including colorectal cancer, where specific microbial imbalances link to inflammation, microbial metabolites, and immune modulation.

9.10.3 The Microbiota-Gut-Immune System Axis: Guardians of Homeostasis

The microbiota-gut-immune system axis is a dynamic partnership responsible for maintaining health. The gut-associated lymphoid tissue (GALT) and mucosal immunity are frontline defenders of homeostasis. Dysbiosis can disrupt this balance, leading to inflammation, immune dysfunction, and an increased risk of cancer.

9.10.4 Influencing Cancer Risk Through Dysbiosis

Evidence suggests that alterations in the gut microbiota elevate the risk of cancer development. Inflammation, microbial metabolites, and gut barrier function are key mechanisms through which the microbiota influences cancer risk. Colorectal cancer, among the most extensively studied, demonstrates a specific connection between bacterial species and cancer risk.

9.10.5 Microbiota in Cancer Treatment: An Evolving Paradigm

Microbiota-based interventions show promise in enhancing cancer treatment outcomes. The microbiota's influence on chemotherapy, immunotherapy, and radiation therapy can improve treatment efficacy and reduce side effects. Probiotics, prebiotics, dietary modifications, and fecal microbiota transplantation offer exciting avenues for optimizing cancer care.

9.10.6 Emerging Research and Challenges: The Promise of Personalized Medicine

Recent research explores microbial signatures linked to different cancer types, stages, and treatment responses. These microbial profiles may guide personalized treatment strategies, yet translating this research into clinical practice faces challenges like patient heterogeneity, resource-intensive trials, and ethical and regulatory considerations.

9.10.7 Modifying Gut Microbiota in Precision Cancer Treatment: An Exciting Frontier

In the context of precision medicine, there is an emerging frontier in modifying gut microbiota dysbiosis. Microbial signatures can guide personalized treatment decisions, potentially improving the effectiveness of cancer therapies. Overcoming challenges and addressing ethical and regulatory considerations are essential for the safe and effective integration of microbiota-based therapies into cancer care.

References

1. Hanahan D, Weinberg RA. Hallmarks of cancer: the next generation. Cell. 2011;144(5):646–74.

2. Yarbro CH, Wujcik D, Gobel BH. Cancer nursing: principles and practice. Burlington, MA: Jones & Bartlett Learning; 2018.
3. Bray F, Ferlay J, Soerjomataram I, Siegel RL, Torre LA, Jemal A. Global cancer statistics 2018: GLOBOCAN estimates of incidence and mortality worldwide for 36 cancers in 185 countries. CA Cancer J Clin. 2018;68(6):394–424.
4. Sullivan R, Peppercorn J, Sikora K, Zalcberg J, Meropol NJ, Amir E, Khayat D, Boyle P, Autier P, Tannock IF, Fojo T, Siderov J, Williamson S, Camporesi S, McVie JG, Purushotham AD, Naredi P, Eggermont A, Brennan MF, Steinberg ML, De Ridder M, McCloskey SA, Verellen D, Roberts T, Storme G, Hicks RJ, Ell PJ, Hirsch BR, Carbone DP, Schulman KA, Catchpole P, Taylor D, Geissler J, Brinker NG, Meltzer D, Kerr D, Aapro M. Delivering affordable cancer care in high-income countries. Lancet Oncol. 2011;12(10):933–80.
5. Sender R, Fuchs S, Milo R. Are we really vastly outnumbered? Revisiting the ratio of bacterial to host cells in humans. Cell. 2016;164(3):337–40.
6. Lloyd-Price J, Abu-Ali G, Huttenhower C. The healthy human microbiome. Genome Med. 2016;8(1):51.
7. Belkaid Y, Hand TW. Role of the microbiota in immunity and inflammation. Cell. 2014;157(1):121–41.
8. Cho I, Blaser MJ. The human microbiome: at the interface of health and disease. Nat Rev Genet. 2012;13(4):260–70.
9. Schwabe RF, Jobin C. The microbiome and cancer. Nat Rev Cancer. 2013;13(11):800–12.
10. Gopalakrishnan V, Helmink BA, Spencer CN, Reuben A, Wargo JA. The influence of the gut microbiome on cancer, immunity, and cancer immunotherapy. Cancer Cell. 2018;33(4):570–80.
11. Thursby E, Juge N. Introduction to the human gut microbiota. Biochem J. 2017;474(11):1823–36.
12. Human Microbiome Project Consortium. Structure, function and diversity of the healthy human microbiome. Nature. 2012;486(7402):207–14.
13. Grice EA, Segre JA. The skin microbiome. Nat Rev Microbiol. 2011;9(4):244–53.
14. Kilian M, Chapple IL, Hannig M, Marsh PD, Meuric V, Pedersen AM, Tonetti MS, Wade WG, Zaura E. The oral microbiome - an update for oral healthcare professionals. Br Dent J. 2016;221(10):657–66.
15. Caporaso JG, Lauber CL, Walters WA, Berg-Lyons D, Huntley J, Fierer N, Owens SM, Betley J, Fraser L, Bauer M, Gormley N, Gilbert JA, Smith G, Knight R. Ultra-high-throughput microbial community analysis on the Illumina HiSeq and MiSeq platforms. ISME J. 2012;6(8):1621–4.
16. Qin J, Li R, Raes J, Arumugam M, Burgdorf KS, Manichanh C, Nielsen T, Pons N, Levenez F, Yamada T, Mende DR, Li J, Xu J, Li S, Li D, Cao J, Wang B, Liang H, Zheng H, Xie Y, Tap J, Lepage P, Bertalan M, Batto JM, Hansen T, Le Paslier D, Linneberg A, Nielsen HB, Pelletier E, Renault P, Sicheritz-Ponten T, Turner K, Zhu H, Yu C, Li S, Jian M, Zhou Y, Li Y, Zhang X, Li S, Qin N, Yang H, Wang J, Brunak S, Doré J, Guarner F, Kristiansen K, Pedersen O, Parkhill J, Weissenbach J; MetaHIT Consortium, Bork P, Ehrlich SD, Wang J. A human gut microbial gene catalogue established by metagenomic sequencing. Nature. 2010;464(7285):59–65.
17. Round JL, Mazmanian SK. The gut microbiota shapes intestinal immune responses during health and disease. Nat Rev Immunol. 2009;9(5):313–23.
18. Hooper LV, Littman DR, Macpherson AJ. Interactions between the microbiota and the immune system. Science. 2012;336(6086):1268–73.
19. Mowat AM, Agace WW. Regional specialization within the intestinal immune system. Nat Rev Immunol. 2014;14(10):667–85.
20. Peterson DA, McNulty NP, Guruge JL, Gordon JI. IgA response to symbiotic bacteria as a mediator of gut homeostasis. Cell Host Microbe. 2007;2(5):328–39.
21. Gagnière J, Raisch J, Veziant J, Barnich N, Bonnet R, Buc E, Bringer MA, Pezet D, Bonnet M. Gut microbiota imbalance and colorectal cancer. World J Gastroenterol. 2016;22(2):501–18.
22. Sears CL, Garrett WS. Microbes, microbiota, and colon cancer. Cell Host Microbe. 2014;15(3):317–28.

23. Arthur JC, Perez-Chanona E, Mühlbauer M, Tomkovich S, Uronis JM, Fan TJ, Campbell BJ, Abujamel T, Dogan B, Rogers AB, Rhodes JM, Stintzi A, Simpson KW, Hansen JJ, Keku TO, Fodor AA, Jobin C. Intestinal inflammation targets cancer-inducing activity of the microbiota. Science. 2012;338(6103):120–3.
24. Mantovani A, Allavena P, Sica A, Balkwill F. Cancer-related inflammation. Nature. 2008;454(7203):436–44.
25. Louis P, Hold GL, Flint HJ. The gut microbiota, bacterial metabolites and colorectal cancer. Nat Rev Microbiol. 2014;12(10):661–72.
26. Fukata M, Shang L, Santaolalla R, Sotolongo J, Pastorini C, España C, Ungaro R, Harpaz N, Cooper HS, Elson G, Kosco-Vilbois M, Zaias J, Perez MT, Mayer L, Vamadevan AS, Lira SA, Abreu MT. Constitutive activation of epithelial TLR4 augments inflammatory responses to mucosal injury and drives colitis-associated tumorigenesis. Inflamm Bowel Dis. 2011;17(11):1464–73.
27. Yu J, Feng Q, Wong SH, Zhang D, Liang QY, Qin Y, Tang L, Zhao H, Stenvang J, Li Y, Wang X, Xu X, Chen N, Wu WK, Al-Aama J, Nielsen HJ, Kiilerich P, Jensen B, Wang J, Liu T, Liu H, Xu X, Qing T, Wu D, Chen Y, Liu Z, Li J, Wang J, Rosenberg J, Brunner N, Jensen L, Ponsaing L, Linneberg A, Guarner F, Pedersen O, Wang J, Bao X, Xu X, Wang J, Yang H, Wang J, Datz C, Du M, Andersen V, Kristiansen K, Brix S, Ehrlich SD, He Y, Li L, Wu M, Yu J, Rieder F, Kassinen A, Bao Q, Nielsen OH, Pedersen O. Metagenomic analysis of faecal microbiome as a tool towards targeted non-invasive biomarkers for colorectal cancer. Gut. 2017;66(1):70–8.
28. Yu LX, Schwabe RF. The gut microbiome and liver cancer: mechanisms and clinical translation. Nat Rev Gastroenterol Hepatol. 2017;14(9):527–39.
29. Thomas RM, Jobin C. Microbiota in pancreatic health and disease: the next frontier in microbiome research. Nat Rev Gastroenterol Hepatol. 2020;17(4):231–40.
30. Ferreira RM, Pereira-Marques J, Pinto-Ribeiro I, Costa JL, Carneiro F, Machado JC, Figueiredo C. Gastric microbial community profiling reveals a dysbiotic cancer-associated microbiota. Gut. 2018;67(2):226–36.
31. Alexander JL, Wilson ID, Teare J, Marchesi JR, Nicholson JK, Kinross JM. Gut microbiota modulation of chemotherapy efficacy and toxicity. Nat Rev Gastroenterol Hepatol. 2017;14(6):356–65.
32. Wallace BD, Wang H, Lane KT, Scott JE, Orans J, Koo JS, Venkatesh M, Jobin C, Yeh LA, Mani S, Redinbo MR. Alleviating cancer drug toxicity by inhibiting a bacterial enzyme. Science. 2010;330(6005):831–5.
33. Routy B, Le Chatelier E, Derosa L, Duong CP, Alou MT, Daillère R, Fluckiger A, Messaoudene M, Rauber C, Roberti MP, Fidelle M, Flament C, Poirier-Colame V, Opolon P, Klein C, Iribarren K, Mondragón L, Jacquelot N, Qu B, Ferrere G, Clémenson C, Mezquita L, Masip JR, Naltet C, Brosseau S, Kaderbhai C, Richard C, Rizvi H, Levenez F, Galleron N, Quinquis B, Pons N, Ryffel B, Minard-Colin V, Gonin P, Soria JC, Deutsch E, Loriot Y, Ghiringhelli F, Zalcman G, Goldwasser F, Escudier B, Hellmann MD, Eggermont A, Raoult D, Albiges L, Kroemer G, Zitvogel L. Gut microbiome influences efficacy of PD-1-based immunotherapy against epithelial tumors. Science. 2018;359(6371):91–7.
34. Dubin K, Callahan MK, Ren B, Khanin R, Viale A, Ling L, No D, Gobourne A, Littmann E, Huttenhower C, Pamer EG, Wolchok JD. Intestinal microbiome analyses identify melanoma patients at risk for checkpoint-blockade-induced colitis. Nat Commun. 2016;7:10391.
35. Van Limbergen EJ, Deboever G, Decraene T, De Leeneer K, Poppe B, Despierre E, Michils G, Trinh XB, Gevaert O, Van Nieuwerburgh F, Bekaert S, Daemen A, Coenegrachts L, Tjalma WA, Lambin P, Vergote I, Nevelstam D, Claes K, Moreau Y, Debruyne PR. Whole exome sequencing of cell-free DNA in an endometrial cancer cohort. BMC Med. 2021;19(1):242.
36. Shui L, Yang X, Li J, Yi C, Sun Q, Zhu H, Wang L, Lai M. Gut microbiome as a potential factor for modulating resistance to cancer immunotherapy. Front Immunol. 2021;11:607149.
37. Mego M, Holec V, Drgona L, Hainova K, Ciernikova S, Zajac V. Probiotic bacteria in cancer patients undergoing chemotherapy and radiation therapy. Complement Ther Med. 2013;21(6):712–23.

38. Kumar M, Nagpal R, Verma V, Kumar A, Kaur N, Hemalatha R, Gautam SK, Singh B, Marotta F, Catanzaro R, Jindal S. Probiotic metabolites as epigenetic targets in the prevention of colon cancer. Nutr Rev. 2013;71(8):23–34.
39. Rafter J, Bennett M, Caderni G, Clune Y, Hughes R, Karlsson PC, Klinder A, O'Riordan M, O'Sullivan GC, Pool-Zobel B, Rechkemmer G, Roller M, Rowland I, Salvadori M, Thijs H, van Loo J. Dietary synbiotics reduce cancer risk factors in polypectomized and colon cancer patients. Am J Clin Nutr. 2007;85(2):488–96.
40. O'Keefe SJ, Li JV, Lahti L, Ou J, Carbonero F, Mohammed K, Posma JM, Kinross J, Wahl E, Ruder E, Vipperla K, Naidoo V, Mtshali L, Tims S, Puylaert PG, DeLany J, Krasinskas A, Benefiel AC, Kaseb HO, Newton K, Nicholson JK, de Vos WM, Gaskins HR, Zoetendal EG. Fat, fibre and cancer risk in African Americans and rural Africans. Nat Commun. 2015;17(6):6342.
41. DeFilipp Z, Peled JU, Li L, Mahabamunuge J, Dagher Z, Slingerland AE, Del Rio C, Valles B, Kempner ME, Smith M, Brown J, Gittelman RM, Weber D, Cotter G, Lehmann L, Heyman B, Ponce DM, O'Reilly RJ, Xavier JB, Satlin MJ, Taur Y, Pamer EG, Jenq RR. Third-party fecal microbiota transplantation following Allo-HCT reconstitutes microbiome diversity. Blood Adv. 2018;2(7):745–53.
42. Louis P, Flint HJ. Formation of propionate and butyrate by the human colonic microbiota. Environ Microbiol. 2017;19(1):29–41.
43. Khoruts A, Sadowsky MJ. Understanding the mechanisms of faecal microbiota transplantation. Nat Rev Gastroenterol Hepatol. 2016;13(9):508–16.

Microbiota and Dermatological Diseases 10

Margarita Sanchez-Pece

10.1 Introduction

The human body is home to a diverse community of microorganisms, known as the microbiota, which includes bacteria, viruses, fungi, and other microbes. The microbiota plays a crucial role in maintaining various aspects of human health, such as digestion, immune function, and protection against pathogens. In recent years, there has been increasing recognition of the microbiota's significance in skin health and its role in dermatological diseases.

10.1.1 Microbiota and Its Significance in Human Health

The microbiota is essential for maintaining homeostasis in the body. Changes to the normal microflora due to genetic or environmental factors can contribute to the development of diseases, including dermatological conditions such as psoriasis, rosacea, and atopic dermatitis. The gut microbiome is thought to play a role in the pathogenesis of atopic dermatitis, and evidence suggests that it may be due to a combination of neurological and immunological factors resulting in chronic systemic inflammation that can ultimately affect the skin [1].

Dysbiosis, or imbalance in the microbiota, has been identified in many dermatological conditions, and microbiota-derived molecules have been linked to changes in the immune system characteristic of several dermatological diseases, especially psoriasis and atopic dermatitis [2].

M. Sanchez-Pece (✉)
Department of Biomedicine, Universidad Alfonso X EL Sabio, Madrid, Spain
e-mail: mvallsan@myuax.com

J. Ruiz-Tovar (ed.), *Dysbiosis*, https://doi.org/10.1007/978-3-031-65650-7_10

10.1.2 Microbiota's Role in Skin Health and Dermatological Diseases

The human skin harbors a wide variety of microbes that form the human skin microbiome. Changes in the cutaneous microbiota are involved in the pathophysiology of several dermatoses, and the skin microbiota can affect human health, with its imbalance and dysbiosis contributing to skin diseases such as acne, psoriasis, and atopic dermatitis [3, 4]. The skin microbiota interacts with epithelial or immune cells and plays critical roles in wound healing, barrier restoration, or pathogenic protection. Quantitative and qualitative changes in the skin microbiota, such as dysbiosis, may closely associate with the dysfunction of the host immune system, possibly leading to the induction of inflammatory disorders [5].

In summary, the microbiota, including the gut and skin microbiome, plays a significant role in human health and is increasingly recognized for its involvement in various dermatological diseases. Understanding the interactions between the microbiota and the skin is important for developing new therapeutic approaches and maintaining skin health. Further research is needed to fully elucidate the mechanisms underlying these interactions and their implications for the diagnosis and treatment of skin conditions.

10.2 The Skin Microbiota

10.2.1 Skin Microbiota Composition and Diversity

The human skin is home to a diverse community of microorganisms, collectively known as the skin microbiota. This microbiota includes bacteria, fungi, and viruses, and its composition and diversity vary across different skin sites. The skin microbiota of a healthy adult remains stable over time, despite environmental perturbations, and its study is valuable for understanding the causes of common skin disorders. The skin microbiota is adapted to utilize the limited nutrients available on the skin and can produce molecules that inhibit the colonization of other microorganisms [6].

Proteobacteria have been found to dominate the skin microbiota at all depths of sampling, and there are strong similarities in the complexity and identity of the skin microbiota between humans and mice [7].

Bacterial diversity on the skin has been found to be high, with interpersonal variation approximately equal to intrapersonal variation. The skin microbiota is also influenced by environmental factors and can be associated with various skin diseases such as acne, psoriasis, and atopic dermatitis [7, 8].

10.2.2 Role of the Skin Microbiota in Maintaining Skin Homeostasis

The skin microbiota plays a crucial role in maintaining skin homeostasis. It interacts with epithelial or immune cells and is involved in wound healing, barrier restoration, and protection against pathogens. Changes in the skin microbiota, such as dysbiosis, have been closely associated with the dysfunction of the host immune system, potentially leading to the development of inflammatory disorders. The skin microbiota's diversity and abundance differ between healthy and diseased states, with many skin diseases being associated with their dysbiosis and imbalance [4, 5].

10.3 Dysbiosis and Skin Health

10.3.1 Dysbiosis and its Impact on the Skin Microbiota

Dysbiosis refers to an imbalance or maladaptation of the microbiota, leading to changes in its composition and function. In the context of the skin microbiota, dysbiosis can result from an overgrowth of pathogenic microorganisms and a decrease in beneficial commensals. This imbalance can lead to various skin diseases, such as acne, eczema, and chronic wounds. Dysbiosis in the skin microbiota is associated with altered immune responses, promoting the development of skin conditions like atopic dermatitis, psoriasis, acne vulgaris, and dandruff [5, 9].

The dysbiosis of the skin microbiota is linked to an increased colonization of pathogens and a decrease in the numbers of beneficial commensals, which can contribute to the pathogenesis of skin diseases [10].

10.3.2 Factors Contributing to Dysbiosis in the Skin

Several factors can contribute to dysbiosis in the skin, including environmental influences, diet, and lifestyle. Environmental factors such as UV radiation, pollution, and temperature can impact the diversity and abundance of the skin microbiota. Additionally, diet and lifestyle choices, such as hygiene practices and the use of antimicrobial agents, can alter the skin microbiota composition. For instance, the use of broad-spectrum antibiotics can disrupt the balance of the skin microbiota, leading to dysbiosis. Furthermore, genetic predisposition and immune system function also play a role in maintaining the balance of the skin microbiota.

Understanding these factors is crucial for managing and preventing dysbiosis-related skin conditions [3, 9].

10.4 Correlation between Microbiota Changes and Dermatological Diseases

10.4.1 Specific Dermatological Diseases Linked to Microbiota Alterations

Several dermatological diseases have been linked to alterations in the skin microbiota, particularly dysbiosis. These include the following:

1. Acne vulgaris: The overgrowth of *Propionibacterium acnes*, a bacterium commonly found on the skin, is associated with the development of acne vulgaris. Changes in the skin microbiota, especially an increase in the population of *P. acnes*, can contribute to the pathogenesis of acne [4].
2. Atopic dermatitis: Alterations in the skin microbiota, including an increase in *Staphylococcus aureus* and a decrease in microbial diversity, have been observed in individuals with atopic dermatitis. These changes can influence the skin's immune responses and contribute to the development and exacerbation of atopic dermatitis [1].
3. Psoriasis: Dysbiosis in the skin microbiota has been implicated in the pathogenesis of psoriasis. The composition and abundance of microorganisms on the skin, particularly bacteria, can influence the immune system and inflammatory responses, potentially contributing to the development of psoriatic lesions [5].

10.4.2 Case Studies and Examples Highlighting the Relationship between Microbiota Changes and Skin Conditions

For instance, research has demonstrated that the overgrowth of certain bacteria, such as *Staphylococcus aureus*, and a decrease in microbial diversity can be associated with the severity of atopic dermatitis [1]. A higher density of *S. aureus* colonization correlates with increased inflammation and more severe AD. Additionally, studies reveal that microbial diversity is compromised in AD, with *Staphylococcus* species dominating, especially *S. aureus*. Reduced microbial diversity contributes to the transition into a diseased state. Protective microorganisms like *S. epidermidis* and *S. cohnii*, promoting microbiome diversity, are linked to a reduced risk of developing eczema. *Firmicutes*, *Bacteroidetes*, and *Streptococcus* increase, while *Actinobacteria* and *Propionibacterium* decrease. Specific strains, like *Xanthomonadaceae*, associated with clinical improvement post-treatment, highlight microbiota's role. Orally administered probiotics positively influence psoriasis, suggesting the potential for accurate molecular signatures for diagnosis [4].

Similarly, studies have shown that the abundance of specific microorganisms, such as *Propionibacterium acnes*, is linked to the pathogenesis of acne vulgaris [4]. One study examined the skin microbiota in acne patients, identifying overabundance of *Proteobacteria* and *Firmicutes*, under-representation of *Actinobacteria*, and increased *Staphylococci* in lesions. Subjects treated with erythromycin or a dermocosmetic showed reduced comedones, papules, and pustules, with both products impacting *Actinobacteria* and *Staphylococci*. Despite topical antibiotic's impact on *Actinobacteria*, *Staphylococcus* remained prevalent genus. The findings suggest both interventions effectively reduce acne lesions, emphasizing the dynamic relationship between skin microbiota and acne development [11].

Rosacea's connection with skin microbiota is less explored than its association with *Demodex* mites. Antibiotics, although effective in treating rosacea, have no impact on *Demodex*, suggesting a potential role for microbes in its pathogenesis. Clinical cases using systemic antibiotics reveal shifts in skin microbiota, such as naturally occurring *S. aureus* and *Corynebacterium bovis* colonization, contributing to inflammation in eczematous dermatitis [4].

These findings highlighted the significant role of the skin microbiota in influencing various dermatological diseases.

10.5 Mechanisms Underlying Microbiota-Skin Interaction

10.5.1 Molecular and Cellular Mechanisms through which the Microbiota Influences Skin Health

The skin microbiota influences skin health through various molecular and cellular mechanisms. The microbiota interacts with the host's immune system, modulates inflammation, and contributes to the maintenance of the skin's barrier function. These interactions are essential for wound healing, pathogen protection, and overall skin homeostasis [5].

The skin microbiota's impact on skin health is mediated by its interactions with epithelial and immune cells. For example, the microbiota can educate the innate and adaptive immune systems, influencing the immune responses mounted by the skin. Additionally, the microbiota contributes to the breakdown of natural products and the production of antimicrobial peptides, which are crucial for protecting the skin from pathogens [6].

10.5.2 Dysbiosis and its Contribution to Inflammation, Immune Responses, and Barrier Function Disruption

Dysbiosis in the skin microbiota can contribute to inflammation, immune responses, and disruption of the skin's barrier function. Alterations in the skin microbiota, such as an overgrowth of pathogenic microorganisms or a decrease in microbial diversity, have been associated with the development and exacerbation of various skin diseases, including atopic dermatitis, psoriasis, acne vulgaris, and dandruff [10].

The dysbiotic skin microbiota can lead to an altered immune response, promoting the development of skin diseases. This altered immune response is linked to changes in the production of antimicrobial peptides, modulation of inflammatory pathways, and impairment of the skin's barrier function. These changes can contribute to the pathogenesis of inflammatory skin disorders [9].

10.6 Therapeutic Implications

10.6.1 Current Therapeutic Interventions Targeting the Skin Microbiota

Current and potential therapeutic interventions targeting the skin microbiota include the use of topical probiotics, prebiotics, and postbiotics for treating various skin disorders. These microbiome-targeted strategies aim to modulate the skin microbiota and improve skin health. However, it is important to note that the use of topical probiotics has been found to have limitations due to insufficient evidence supporting their effectiveness [12].

Additionally, the administration of specific bacterial strains has been investigated as a potential bacteriotherapy for inflammatory skin diseases, although the safety, efficacy, and sustainability of this therapeutic approach using isolated live bacteria need further evaluation [13].

Probiotics, prebiotics, and other microbiota-modulating approaches are being explored for managing dermatological diseases by targeting the skin microbiota. Probiotics, which are live microorganisms that confer a health benefit to the host, have been studied for their potential in modulating the skin microbiota and immune responses, offering therapeutic benefits for conditions such as atopic dermatitis, psoriasis, and acne vulgaris [14, 15].

Prebiotics, on the other hand, are substances that promote the growth and activity of beneficial microorganisms and are being investigated for their ability to support a healthy skin microbiota and improve skin conditions [14].

10.6.2 Applications

Probiotics, prebiotics, and antimicrobial peptides have potential applications in maintaining or restoring the skin microbiome.

Probiotics, such as *Lactobacillus* and *Bifidobacterium*, have been suggested as adjunctive treatments for dermatological diseases like atopic dermatitis or acne. These beneficial bacteria can help restore the balance of the skin microbiome, promoting a healthy environment.

Prebiotics, which serve as food for beneficial bacteria, can also be used to support the growth and activity of these bacteria, aiding in the restoration of the skin microbiome.

Additionally, antimicrobial peptides (AMPs) expressed by the skin can play a role in maintaining the microbiome's homeostasis by providing a defense against pathogenic microbial stimuli. These peptides are effective against a variety of microbial skin colonizers, including bacteria and fungi, and may offer a potential future treatment option for inflammatory skin diseases caused by pathogens.

These applications align with the concept of ecobiology, which focuses on maintaining or restoring the skin microbiome's homeostasis to protect the body from external aggressions and infections. By utilizing suitable topical products with a pH close to that of the skin and incorporating probiotics, prebiotics, and AMPs, it may be possible to support the health and balance of the skin microbiome [16].

10.7 Future Directions and Challenges

Ongoing research and emerging trends in understanding the microbiota-skin connection are focused on several key areas, as highlighted in the provided sources:

1. Microbial Identification: Traditional microbial research has focused on understanding the interactions between the skin microbiota and the host. However, challenges persist in accurately identifying and characterizing the diverse microorganisms that comprise the skin microbiota. Culture-independent methods, such as high-throughput sequencing, have expanded our understanding of the skin microbiome's role in maintaining health or promoting disease. However, not all skin microbes are necessarily recoverable via culture, leading to potential underestimation of microbial diversity [17, 18].
2. Modeling the Skin Microbiome: Another area of research involves the development of models to better understand the dynamics of the skin microbiome. This includes investigating the specific associations between the skin's physiology and its microbiome, as well as the competitive and synergistic interactions between microorganisms and the host. These efforts aim to elucidate the complex relationships within the skin microbiota and their implications for skin health and disease [18].
3. Therapeutic Interventions: Research is also focused on exploring the association of the skin microbiota with various skin disorders and developing therapeutic interventions. This includes investigating the implications of cosmetics on the skin microbiome and studying the potential of rebiosis (restoring microbial balance) as a therapeutic approach for conditions such as atopic dermatitis, psoriasis, and acne vulgaris [14].

Challenges and gaps in knowledge that require further exploration include the need to overcome limitations in microbial identification, establish a comprehensive understanding of the skin microbiome's composition and function in health and disease, and develop effective therapeutic interventions that target the skin microbiota. Additionally, understanding the specific associations between the skin's physiology and its microbiome, as well as the complex interactions within the skin microbiota, remains a key challenge in advancing our knowledge of the microbiota-skin connection [17, 18].

10.8 Conclusions

In conclusion, the microbiota's role in dermatological diseases is crucial, emphasizing its significance in maintaining skin health. Dysbiosis, characterized by microbial imbalances, plays a critical role in skin disorders like psoriasis, rosacea, and atopic dermatitis. The skin microbiota, pivotal for wound healing and immune modulation, is influenced by various factors, contributing to inflammatory responses when disrupted.

Exploring specific dermatological diseases, such as acne vulgaris and psoriasis, reveals correlations between microbiota alterations and disease severity. Case studies highlight the importance of microbial diversity in clinical outcomes.

Examining molecular mechanisms, we uncover how the microbiota influences immune responses, inflammation, and skin barrier function. Therapeutic interventions, from current strategies like topical probiotics to emerging bacteriotherapies, offer avenues for managing dysbiosis-related skin conditions. Challenges persist in microbial identification and therapeutic efficacy, necessitating ongoing research.

Navigating future directions, integrating microbiota analysis into dermatological diagnostics promises personalized treatments. The quest for a comprehensive understanding of the skin microbiome's role in health and disease, along with ethical considerations and therapeutic innovations, outlines the dynamic relationship between microbiota and skin health. This journey provides a foundation for advancing dermatological research and personalized treatment approaches.

References

1. Ellis SR, Nguyen M, Vaughn AR, Notay M, Burney WA, Sandhu S, et al. The skin and gut microbiome and its role in common dermatologic conditions. Microorganisms. 2019;7(11):550.
2. Stec A, Sikora M, Maciejewska M, Paralusz-Stec K, Michalska M, Sikorska E, et al. Bacterial metabolites: a link between gut microbiota and dermatological diseases. Int J Mol Sci. 2023;24(4):3494. https://pubmed.ncbi.nlm.nih.gov/36834904/
3. Carmona-Cruz S, Orozco-Covarrubias L, Sáez-de-Ocariz M. The human skin microbiome in selected cutaneous diseases. Front Cell Infect Microbiol. 2022;12:834135. https://doi.org/10.3389/fcimb.2022.834135.
4. Yang Y, Qu L, Mijakovic I, Wei Y. Advances in the human skin microbiota and its roles in cutaneous diseases. Microb Cell Factories. 2022;21(1):176. Available from: https://doi.org/10.1186/s12934-022-01901-6
5. Park EJ, Yadav H, Singh TP. Editorial: microbiota in skin inflammatory diseases. Front Immunol. 2023;14:1235314. https://doi.org/10.3389/fimmu.2023.1235314.
6. Byrd AL, Belkaid Y, Segre JA. The human skin microbiome. Nat Rev Microbiol. 2018;16(3):143–55. https://www.nature.com/articles/nrmicro.2017.157
7. Grice EA, Kong HH, Renaud G, Young AC, Bouffard GG, Blakesley RW, et al. A diversity profile of the human skin microbiota. Genome Res. 2008;18(7):1043–50. https://doi.org/10.1101/gr.075549.107.
8. Suwarsa O, Hazari MN, Dharmadji HP, Dwiyana RF, Effendi RMRA, Hidayah RMN, et al. A pilot study: composition and diversity of 16S rRNA based skin bacterial microbiome in Indonesian atopic dermatitis population. Clin Cosmet Investig Dermatol. 2021;14:1737–44.

https://www.dovepress.com/a-pilot-study-composition-and-diversity-of-16s-rrna-based-skin-bacteri-peer-reviewed-fulltext-article-CCID

9. Liang X, Ou C, Zhuang J, Li J, Zhang F, Zhong Y, et al. Interplay between skin microbiota dysbiosis and the host immune system in psoriasis: potential pathogenesis. Front Immunol. 2021;12:764384. https://doi.org/10.3389/fimmu.2021.764384.
10. De Pessemier B, Grine L, Debaere M, Maes A, Paetzold B, Callewaert C. Gut–skin axis: current knowledge of the interrelationship between microbial dysbiosis and skin conditions. Microorganisms. 2021;9(2):353. https://doi.org/10.3390/microorganisms9020353.
11. Dreno B, Martin R, Moyal D, Henley JB, Khammari A, Seité S. Skin microbiome and *acne vulgaris*: *staphylococcus*, a new actor in acne. Exp Dermatol. 2017;26(9):798–803. https://pubmed.ncbi.nlm.nih.gov/28094874/
12. AL-Smadi K, Leite-Silva VR, Filho NA, Lopes PS, Mohammed Y. Innovative approaches for maintaining and enhancing skin health and managing skin diseases through microbiome-targeted strategies. Antibiotics (Basel). 2023;12(12):1698. https://www.mdpi.com/2079-6382/12/12/1698
13. Ito Y, Amagai M. Controlling skin microbiome as a new bacteriotherapy for inflammatory skin diseases. Inflamm Regen. 2022;42(1):26. https://doi.org/10.1186/s41232-022-00212-y.
14. Seethalakshmi PS, Hassan S, Kiran GS, Bramhachari PV, Selvin J. The dynamics of skin microbiome: Association of Microbiota with skin disorders and therapeutic intervention. In: Human microbiome in health, disease, and therapy. Singapore: Springer Nature; 2023. p. 187–204.
15. Grice E. The skin microbiome: potential for novel diagnostic and therapeutic approaches to cutaneous disease. Semin Cutan Med Surg. 2014;33(2):98–103. https://doi.org/10.12788/j.sder.0087.
16. Dréno B. The microbiome, a new target for ecobiology in dermatology. Eur J Dermatol. 2019;29(S1):15–8. https://doi.org/10.1684/ejd.2019.3535.
17. Santiago-Rodriguez TM, Le François B, Macklaim JM, Doukhanine E, Hollister EB. The skin microbiome: current techniques, challenges, and future directions. Microorganisms. 2023;11(5):1222. https://doi.org/10.3390/microorganisms11051222.
18. Smythe P, Wilkinson HN. The skin microbiome: current landscape and future opportunities. Int J Mol Sci. 2023;24(4):3950. https://www.mdpi.com/1422–0067/24/4/3950.

11 Microbiota and Ageing

María-Encarnación Fernández-Contreras

11.1 Introduction

The World Health Organization (WHO) has defined healthy ageing as *the process of developing and maintaining the functional ability that enables well-being in older age.*

Functional ability means having the capabilities to enable people to be and do what they value. It is referred to as the ability [1]:

- To meet their basic needs.
- To learn, grow and make decisions.
- To be mobile.
- To build and maintain relationships.
- To contribute to society.

At the biological level, ageing results from the impact of the accumulation of a wide variety of molecular and cellular damage over time. This leads to a gradual decrease in physical and mental capacity, a growing risk of disease and, eventually, death.

Older age is also characterized by the emergence of several complex health states commonly called geriatric syndromes. They are often the consequence of multiple underlying factors and include frailty, urinary incontinence, falls, delirium and pressure ulcers.

Health conditions commonly associated with age include neurodegenerative, cardiovascular or musculoskeletal disorders, as well as diabetes, most of them sharing an inflammatory/immunological component. This led to the creation of a new term: "inflamm-ageing" or "inflammageing", defined as an age-related increase in

M.-E. Fernández-Contreras (✉)
School of Medicine, Universidad Alfonso X el Sabio, Villanueva de la Cañada, Madrid, Spain

J. Ruiz-Tovar (ed.), *Dysbiosis*, https://doi.org/10.1007/978-3-031-65650-7_11

the levels of blood and tissue pro-inflammatory markers [2]. As people age, they are more likely to experience several conditions at the same time.

Gut microbiota has gained increasing relevance among the multiple factors related with age. Recent research points out to an impact on human health and ageing processes. Dysbiosis is a risk factor for age-related diseases, but, in contrast, the presence of a wide variety of microbial taxa has been claimed to increase life expectancy. Indeed, significant differences in the composition of gut microbiota between centenarians and younger elderly have been reported [3, 4].

Hence, microbiota might play a key role in the so-called healthy ageing, and, more interestingly, it is emerging as a promising target for anti-ageing therapies.

11.2 Evolution of Microbiota and Physiological and Functional Changes in the Elderly's Gastrointestinal Tract

Microbiota acquirement occurs early in life. In fact, it was thought that the foetus was sterile *in utero*, and the new-born was colonized during delivery, but recent studies revealed that such colonization takes place during pregnancy [5]. Commensal bacteria have been detected in meconium, placenta, and umbilical cord of healthy new-borns, even upon aseptic caesarean section [6]. Moreover, inoculation of pregnant mice with labelled *Enterococcus faecium* isolated from human breastmilk has shown transmission from the mother's gastrointestinal tract to amniotic fluid that is eventually swallowed by the foetus [5, 7].

The composition of this primary microbiota is influenced by a number of factors, including mode of delivery (vaginal vs. caesarean birth), early feeding (breast vs. formula) as well as antibiotic treatment, maternal diet, or environment [8]. During vaginal delivery, the new-born is exposed to the microbiome of the mother's birth canal, whereas, in the case of caesarean birth, he will be exposed to her skin. As a result, the microbiota of naturally delivered infants is like that of the mother's vaginal canal, while that of children born by caesarean section resembles that of the mother's skin [5, 9]. In addition, caesarean-born infants are also subjected to longer hospital stays, or antibiotic therapy, which may contribute to differences with vaginally delivered ones [8].

Regarding early feeding, breast-fed babies have more bifidobacteria, lactobacilli, staphylococci and streptococci, while those fed with formula show increased populations of *Bacteroides*, clostridia and proteobacteria [8]. Similarities between breast-fed infant and mother's gut microbiota are explained by bacterial translocation and transport to the mammary gland by dendritic cells [10, 11].

Once established, the microbiota gets relatively stable after weaning. Thereafter, diet will be the major factor affecting the maintenance of gut microbiota composition [5, 8] until the elderly, where its composition changes. This shift of microbial diversity has been linked to age functional impairment, although it remains unclear whether these changes are the cause or the consequence of the ageing processes.

Overall, there is a decrease in beneficial commensals (*Bacteroides*, bifidobacteria, lactobacilli, or genera like *Coprococcus* or *Faecalibacterium*) and an increase in opportunistic pathogens, such as enterobacteria or clostridia [8, 12]. There is also a reduction in the species diversity and population of *Bacteroides*, a genus key in the metabolism of most polysaccharides in the colon [13].

As mentioned above, the main factor determining changes in the composition and balance of intestinal microbiota is diet. In turn, diet in the elderly is directly affected by physiological and functional factors, including decline in taste and smell, loss of teeth or swallowing difficulties. It is well known that the senses of taste and smell are progressive depressed with age, making foods tasteless and unappetizing for geriatric patients. This results in a decline of appetite, which may lead to malnutrition [13, 14], and/or in excessive intake of sugar and salt, causing dental problems like denture-related stomatitis, or periodontal disease [14] that may lead to tooth loss. Consequently, chewing function is dramatically impaired. Also, age-associated sarcopenia has been shown to affect the muscled involved in swallowing [15]. All these factors lead to a limited and imbalanced diet that directly impacts on microbiota.

Bowel function is a key factor that directly determines shifts in bacterial population. Age-related changes like loss of rectal elasticity or reduced muscle tone of the anal internal sphincter, coupled with a decrease of the physical activity and the effect of the medications frequently used by elderly, result in a significant impairment in gut motility, eventually leading to constipation [16]. In turn, slow intestinal transit is related with putrefactive processes in the colon caused by increased protein fermentation by proteolytic bacteria [13, 17], which have been reported to increase in the elderly [8]. As a result, there is a raise in harmful metabolites such as ammonia, indoles or phenols that predispose older people to diseases, as well as to infections by clostridia, especially after antibiotherapy. The impact on the composition of microbiota of the above-mentioned changes in bowel function may explain the dramatic differences between patients in long-term residential care and old adults living in the community [8, 18].

11.3 Microbiota and Immunity: Inflammageing

The term "inflamm-ageing" was first coined in by Franceschi et al. in 2000 [2]. It may be defined as an age-related condition characterized by increased levels of inflammatory markers that predisposes to chronic morbidity, disability, frailty, and premature death [12]. These authors consider that the major characteristics of this phenomenon are a global reduction in the capacity to cope with a variety of stressors and a concomitant progressive increase in proinflammatory status. They also state that the ageing process is indirectly controlled by defence functions or anti-stress responses to physical, chemical, and biological agents (the latter including viruses and bacteria), claiming that immune and stress responses are equivalent. Hence, antigens are nothing but a particular type of stressor [2]. In line with this, levels of age-associated pro-inflammatory markers are increased in the majority of older adults, even in the absence of risk factors and/or clinically active diseases [12].

The ageing process is caused by a prolonged exposition to stress and antigenic load. Consequently, the persistence of inflammatory stimuli over time represents the first hit favouring the susceptibility to age-related conditions associated with inflammation. Hence, inflammageing represents a risk factor for multiple age-associated chronic diseases such as Alzheimer's disease and other neurodegenerative conditions, atherosclerosis, sarcopenia and osteoporosis, diabetes or cancer, among others.

In this line, one of the morphological alterations associated with gut ageing is the changes in shape, size and allocation of intestinal follicles [19], which may constitute the anatomical expression of an altered immune function. The gastrointestinal tract is the largest immunological organ in the body, playing a key role in the regulation of immune homeostasis. In fact, the GI tract might harbour up to 70% of the body's lymphocyte population. Moreover, it is the largest interface in contact with the external environment and a major line of defence [20]. Therefore, an impaired intestinal function parallels with an impaired immune function.

Ageing is associated with a reduction in beneficial commensal, such as *Coprococcus*, *Faecalibacterium*, or *Lactobacillus*, as well as a decrease in the *Firmicutes*/*Bacteroidetes* ratio, which has been reported in inflammatory conditions as IBD [21]. Importantly, a decline in the number and species diversity of *Bacteroides* with age has also been reported. Besides counteracting the expansion of pathogens, these commensals produce mucus and metabolites like short-chain fatty acids (SCFA), which have shown to improve intestinal barrier function [12, 22]. Among them, the genus *Bacteroidetes* may account for the digestion of most polysaccharides in the colon because it can use a wide variety of carbon sources [13]. Meanwhile, the population of other bacteria, mainly facultative anaerobes (e.g. genera *Fusobacterium*, *Clostridium* or *Staphylococcus*), increases in the elderly and may became pathogenic under altered immunological states [8, 12, 13, 19].

In contrast, dysbiosis contributes to reduced gut epithelial integrity through the disruption of tight junctions [22, 23]. Gastrointestinal epithelium constitutes a physical barrier where intestinal epithelial cells (IEC) are strongly involved in innate immunity. An essential piece of such barrier are tight junction complexes, that create a seal between adjacent IECs. Under normal circumstances, there is a dynamic control of tight junction components to prevent the entry of pathogens while regulating permeability to water, ions and nutrients. In contrast, dysregulation in the expression of tight junction components severely affects the barrier function [20]. As a result, a variety of microorganisms and microbial factors like pathogen-associated molecular patterns and damage-associated molecular patterns (PAMPs and DAMPs) are able to pass through into host cells and into the bloodstream [12, 24], thus raising the load of the antigen/stressors referred by Franceschi et al. [2] and, subsequently, the inflammatory response.

11.4 Gut Microbiota of Centenarians

During the first decade of this century, the possibility that the gut microbiota composition could either affect or be affected by the ageing process has gained attention among researchers. Most studies agree that there is a decrease in gut microbial diversity, together with an increase of opportunistic pathogens, such as streptococci, staphylococci, enterobacteria and enterococci. As mentioned above, there is also a decline in beneficial commensals, accompanied by rearrangements in the saccharolytic and proteolytic bacteria (e.g. decrease in the *Firmicutes/Bacteroidetes* ratio) with a decline in SCFA producers [3, 4, 12, 13, 22].

However, studies performed in older individuals must deal with the inconvenience of a high interindividual variability, due the high frequency of comorbidities, the subsequent exposure to multiple medications and a variety of dietary habits and lifestyle [3].

An example is the research run by Biagi et al. [25]. In order to identify what they call a "signature" of extreme ageing in bowel microbiota, the authors defined a group of young (mean age, 30 years), a group of "young elderly" (aged 65–75 years) and a group of "long-living" subjects, in turn subdivided into centenarians (99–104 years old) and semi-supercentenarians (105–109 years old), all enrolled in the same, delimited geographic area in Italy. They found that, despite sharing the characteristics of an elderly-type gut microbiota (decrease in saccharolytic butyrate producers, increase in possibly opportunistic bacteria), that of centenarians and, especially, semi-supercentenarians showed an unexpected increase in bacteria such as *Christensenellaceae*, *Akkermansia* or *Bifidobacterium*, related to good immunological and metabolic status.

In addition, and with the aim of determining microbiota changes strictly associated to longevity, excluding biases due to lifestyle, environment and/or diet, they used bioinformatics and sequencing tools to reanalyse data from the microbiome of Italian and Japanese centenarians (>95 years old) and younger adults from two different studies performed in Italian [25] and Japanese individuals [26]. As mentioned elsewhere, diet is the major factor determining changes in the microbiota, and there are marked differences between Mediterranean diet, rich in whole cereals, fish, vegetables, fruit and olive oil, and the Japanese diet characterized by a high consumption of refined rice, soy-derived foods, fish, fruit and vegetables, but much lower intake of energy and oils/fats. Nevertheless, their results showed that the microbiota of extreme aged adults of both groups shared features as relative abundance of single genera and increase or decrease of determined bacterial groups with a trend to a decline in the impact of lifestyle and environmental variables.

Other studies support that the composition of the gut microbiota of centenarians is similar to that of young adults and has the faculty of promoting anti-inflammatory and antioxidant actions, which are able to counteract the processes leading to age-related diseases [4]. Moreover, it has been reported that there is up-regulation of genes involved in glycolysis and SCFA production.

11.5 Healthy Ageing

The WHO has defined healthy ageing as *the process of developing and maintaining the functional ability that enables well-being in older age* [1]. Functional ability refers to the capabilities that enables people to be and do what they value, i.e.:

- Meet their basic needs.
- Learn, grow and make decisions.
- Be mobile.
- Build and maintain relationships.
- Contribute to society.

In addition, functional ability consists of the interactions between the intrinsic capacity of the individual and relevant environmental characteristics.

In turn, intrinsic capacity comprises all the mental and physical capacities that a person can employ, including his/her ability to walk, think, see, hear and remember, and it is influenced by various factors such as the presence of diseases or age-related changes.

The WHO also sets two key considerations for healthy ageing: diversity that implies that there is not a typical elderly, so that dramatic differences in terms of physical and mental status are found between old adults with the same age, and inequity that refers to the variability of environmental, social and demographic factors (sex, ethnicity, level of education, economical and familiar status) and their impact on people's lives, thereby determining diversity.

As the ageing of the global population has become the most relevant medical and social demographic problem worldwide, the WHO has implementing specific programs to address it, and, basing on previous actions, the decade of 2020–2030 has been established as the decade of Healthy Ageing [1, 27].

11.6 Microbiota and Interventions for Healthy Ageing

Given that evidence strongly suggests a link between gut microbiota and inflammatory age-related disorders (inflammageing), it could be also a putative target to ameliorate the ageing process.

The association between a characteristic composition of microbiota and healthy ageing was already suggested by Elie Metchnikoff, in the early 1900s [8, 13, 28, 29]. He observed that Bulgarian farmers, who routinely consumed large amounts of fermented milk derivatives, were long-lived and attributed their longevity to a beneficial effect of the live microbes. Upon his findings, he distinguished two types of metabolism for gut bacteria: proteolytic that leads to putrefaction and to the production of harmful metabolites ("autotoxins") and saccharolytic (fermentative), with beneficial health-promoting end-products.

Metchnikoff termed this process as "autointoxication" and hypothesized that the primary cause of age-related illnesses is the immune response of reactive phagocytes to the autotoxins generated in the proteolytic/putrefactive events that take place in the bowel, and that restoring gut microflora by regularly consuming yogurt could promote healthier ageing. Moreover, he postulated that the metabolism of fermentative, particularly lactic bacteria could counteract the putrefactive processes of proteolytic ones [8]. Metchnikoff was laureated with the Nobel Prize, that he shared with Paul Ehrlich, in 1908.

Basing on Metchnikoff's theories, in the early 1930s, the Japanese microbiologist Minoru Shirota cultured and isolated the first probiotic bacterium: *Lactobacillus casei Shirota*, a strain of *Lactobacillus casei* that he used to develop a beverage of fermented milk that he called Yakult [29].

Despite these early findings, the impact of intestinal microbiota on human health did not start to gain interest until relatively recent years, when the use of microorganism-based dietary products has started to be considered as potential tool to improve health and delay age-related alterations [8].

In order to favour the development of beneficial bacteria by modifying the composition of gut microbiota, various methods have been proposed, the most relevant being probiotics, prebiotics and symbiotics [4].

Probiotics are defined as live microbial feed which beneficially affects the intestinal microbial balance, prebiotics are non-digestible foods that improve the growth of bacteria in the colon, and symbiotics or eubiotics are mixtures of probiotics and prebiotics [30]. More recently, the concept of "postbiotics" defined as "a preparation of inanimate microorganisms and/or their components that confers a health benefit on the host" was also introduced [31], and their potential benefits for human health are under study.

Fermentation of prebiotics by probiotics, mainly bifidobacteria and lactobacilli, also increases the intestinal levels of SCFAs especially butyrate which, as mentioned earlier, confer immune-modulating and anti-inflammatory effects and contribute to the maintenance of the intestinal barrier of gut barrier [8].

Studies in animal models showed the efficacy of probiotics in restoring the immune system homeostasis and reducing the levels of proinflammatory markers, as well as various positive physiological effects (memory reinforcement, improving neuronal and synaptic lesions, bone mass increment), although results in humans are still inconclusive [4].

More recently, faecal transplantation has also been used as a tool for complete repopulation of the gut microbiota. It consists of a colonic lavage to remove the resident microbial community, followed by the infusion of a suspension of faeces from a donor, during endoscopy or colonoscopy. This approach seems to be promising in cases of patients with recurrent infections by *Clostridioides difficile* that are refractory to antibiotics [32, 33].

11.7 Conclusions

Once gut microbiota is stabilized, the major factor affecting its composition is diet. In the elderly, diet is affected by functional factors like impaired taste and smell and difficulties for chewing and swallowing. This circumstance, together with morphological and functional age-related changes in the intestine, determines a pronounce shift in the configuration of the elderly microbiota, which derives in a characteristic inflammatory status (inflammaging).

The notable differences found between the microbial gut population of centenarians and that of old adults, as well as the observation that many of them consume fermented dairy products have led to the research and development of strategies directed to the gut microbiota as a potential therapeutic target.

Although further, preferably large-scale studies are needed to ascertain the efficacy of interventions with probiotics, prebiotics or symbiotics, as well as other strategies like faecal transplantation, in the case of some refractory intestinal infections, these approaches seem to be promising in order to delay or counteract the processes related with aging.

References

1. https://www.who.int/news-room/questions-and-answers/item/healthy-ageing-and-functional-ability#
2. Franceschi C, Bonafè M, Valensin S, Olivieri F, De Luca M, Ottaviani E, De Benedictis G, Inflamm-aging. An evolutionary perspective on immunosenescence. Ann N Y Acad Sci. 2000;908:244–54. https://doi.org/10.1111/j.1749-6632.2000.tb06651.x.
3. Biagi E, Rampelli S, Turroni S, Quercia S, Candela M, Brigidi P. The gut microbiota of centenarians: signatures of longevity in the gut microbiota profile. Mech Ageing Dev. 2016;165(Pt B):180–4. https://doi.org/10.1016/j.mad.2016.12.013.
4. Salazar J, Durán P, Díaz MP, Chacín M, Santeliz R, Mengual E, Gutiérrez E, León X, Díaz A, Bernal M, Escalona D, Hernández LAP, Bermúdez V. Exploring the relationship between the gut microbiota and ageing: a possible age modulator. Int J Environ Res Public Health. 2023;20(10):5845. https://doi.org/10.3390/ijerph20105845.
5. Lynch DB, Jeffery IB, O'Toole PW. The role of the microbiota in ageing: current state and perspectives. Wiley Interdiscip Rev Syst Biol Med. 2015;7(3):131–8. https://doi.org/10.1002/wsbm.1293.
6. Jiménez E, Fernández L, Marín ML, Martín R, Odriozola JM, Nueno-Palop C, Narbad A, Olivares M, Xaus J, Rodríguez JM. Isolation of commensal bacteria from umbilical cord blood of healthy neonates born by cesarean section. Curr Microbiol. 2005;51(4):270–4. https://doi.org/10.1007/s00284-005-0020-3.
7. Jiménez E, Marín ML, Martín R, Odriozola JM, Olivares M, Xaus J, Fernández L, Rodríguez JM. Is meconium from healthy newborns actually sterile? Res Microbiol. 2008;159(3):187–93. https://doi.org/10.1016/j.resmic.2007.12.007.
8. Nagpal R, Mainali R, Ahmadi S, Wang S, Singh R, Kavanagh K, Kitzman DW, Kushugulova A, Marotta F, Yadav H. Gut microbiome and aging: physiological and mechanistic insights. Nutr Healthy Aging. 2018;4(4):267–85. https://doi.org/10.3233/NHA-170030.
9. Dominguez-Bello MG, Costello EK, Contreras M, Magris M, Hidalgo G, Fierer N, Knight R. Delivery mode shapes the acquisition and structure of the initial microbiota across mul-

tiple body habitats in newborns. Proc Natl Acad Sci USA. 2010;107(26):11971–5. https://doi.org/10.1073/pnas.1002601107.
10. Fernández L, Langa S, Martín V, Jiménez E, Martín R, Rodríguez JM. The microbiota of human milk in healthy women. Cell Mol Biol (Noisy-le-Grand). 2013;59(1):31–42.
11. Donnet-Hughes A, Perez PF, Doré J, Leclerc M, Levenez F, Benyacoub J, Serrant P, Segura-Roggero I, Schiffrin EJ. Potential role of the intestinal microbiota of the mother in neonatal immune education. Proc Nutr Soc. 2010;69(3):407–15. https://doi.org/10.1017/S0029665110001898.
12. Ferrucci L, Fabbri E. Inflammageing: chronic inflammation in ageing, cardiovascular disease, and frailty. Nat Rev Cardiol. 2018;15(9):505–22. https://doi.org/10.1038/s41569-018-0064-2.
13. Woodmansey EJ. Intestinal bacteria and ageing. J Appl Microbiol. 2007;102(5):1178–86. https://doi.org/10.1111/j.1365-2672.2007.03400.x.
14. Winkler S, Garg AK, Mekayarajjananonth T, Bakaeen LG, Khan E. Depressed taste and smell in geriatric patients. J Am Dent Assoc. 1999;130(12):1759–65. https://doi.org/10.14219/jada.archive.1999.0133.
15. Christmas C, Rogus-Pulia N. Swallowing disorders in the older population. J Am Geriatr Soc. 2019;67(12):2643–9. https://doi.org/10.1111/jgs.16137.
16. Mari A, Mahamid M, Amara H, Baker FA, Yaccob A. Chronic constipation in the elderly patient: updates in evaluation and management. Korean J Fam Med. 2020;41(3):139–45. https://doi.org/10.4082/kjfm.18.0182.
17. Macfarlane GT, Cummings JH, Macfarlane S, Gibson GR. Influence of retention time on degradation of pancreatic enzymes by human colonic bacteria grown in a 3-stage continuous culture system. J Appl Bacteriol. 1989;67(5):520–7.
18. Claesson MJ, Jeffery IB, Conde S, Power SE, O'Connor EM, Cusack S, Harris HM, Coakley M, Lakshminarayanan B, O'Sullivan O, Fitzgerald GF, Deane J, O'Connor M, Harnedy N, O'Connor K, O'Mahony D, van Sinderen D, Wallace M, Brennan L, Stanton C, Marchesi JR, Fitzgerald AP, Shanahan F, Hill C, Ross RP, O'Toole PW. Gut microbiota composition correlates with diet and health in the elderly. Nature. 2012;488(7410):178–84. https://doi.org/10.1038/nature11319.
19. Ribera Casado JM. Microbiota intestinal y envejecimiento: ¿un nuevo camino de intervención? [Intestinal microbiota and ageing: A new intervention route?]. Rev Esp Geriatr Gerontol. 2016;51(5):290–5. Spanish. https://doi.org/10.1016/j.regg.2015.12.012.
20. Takiishi T, Fenero CIM, Câmara NOS. Intestinal barrier and gut microbiota: shaping our immune responses throughout life. Tissue Barriers. 2017;5(4):e1373208. https://doi.org/10.1080/21688370.2017.1373208.
21. Stojanov S, Berlec A, Štrukelj B. The influence of probiotics on the firmicutes/Bacteroidetes ratio in the treatment of obesity and inflammatory bowel disease. Microorganisms. 2020;8(11):1715. https://doi.org/10.3390/microorganisms8111715.
22. Pohl K, Moodley P, Dhanda A. The effect of increasing intestinal short-chain fatty acid concentration on gut permeability and liver injury in the context of liver disease: a systematic review. J Gastroenterol Hepatol. 2022;37(8):1498–506. https://doi.org/10.1111/jgh.15899.
23. Wang F, Li Q, He Q, Geng Y, Tang C, Wang C, Li J. Temporal variations of the ileal microbiota in intestinal ischemia and reperfusion. Shock. 2013;39(1):96–103. https://doi.org/10.1097/SHK.0b013e318279265f.
24. Li Q, Zhang Q, Wang C, Li N, Li J. Invasion of enteropathogenic Escherichia coli into host cells through epithelial tight junctions. FEBS J. 2008;275(23):6022–32. https://doi.org/10.1111/j.1742-4658.2008.06731.x.
25. Biagi E, Franceschi C, Rampelli S, Severgnini M, Ostan R, Turroni S, Consolandi C, Quercia S, Scurti M, Monti D, Capri M, Brigidi P, Candela M. Gut microbiota and extreme longevity. Curr Biol. 2016;26(11):1480–5. https://doi.org/10.1016/j.cub.2016.04.016.
26. Odamaki T, Kato K, Sugahara H, Hashikura N, Takahashi S, Xiao JZ, Abe F, Osawa R. Age-related changes in gut microbiota composition from newborn to centenarian: a cross-sectional study. BMC Microbiol. 2016;16:90. https://doi.org/10.1186/s12866-016-0708-5.

27. Wu L, Zeng T, Zinellu A, Rubino S, Kelvin DJ, Carru C. A cross-sectional study of compositional and functional profiles of gut microbiota in Sardinian centenarians. mSystems. 2019;4(4):e00325–19. https://doi.org/10.1128/mSystems.00325-19.
28. Rudnicka E, Napierała P, Podfigurna A, Męczekalski B, Smolarczyk R, Grymowicz M. The World Health Organization (WHO) approach to healthy ageing. Maturitas. 2020;139:6–11. https://doi.org/10.1016/j.maturitas.2020.05.018.
29. Metchnikoff E. The prolongation of life. Optimistic Studies. Putnam's Son. New York and London: The Knickerbocker press; 1908. http://archive.org/stream/prolongationofli00metcuoft#page/14/mode/2up
30. Brüssow H. Microbiota and healthy ageing: observational and nutritional intervention studies. Microb Biotechnol. 2013;6(4):326–34. https://doi.org/10.1111/1751-7915.12048.
31. Zoppi G. Probiotici, prebiotici, sinbiotici ed eubiotici [Probioticss, prebiotics, synbiotics and eubiotics]. Pediatr Med Chir. 1998;20(1):13–7. Italian
32. Vinderola G, Sanders ME, Salminen S. The concept of postbiotics. Foods. 2022;11(8):1077. https://doi.org/10.3390/foods11081077.
33. Lemon KP, Armitage GC, Relman DA, Fischbach MA. Microbiota-targeted therapies: an ecological perspective. Sci Transl Med. 2012;4(137):137rv5. https://doi.org/10.1126/scitranslmed.3004183.
34. Gough E, Shaikh H, Manges AR. Systematic review of intestinal microbiota transplantation (fecal bacteriotherapy) for recurrent Clostridium difficile infection. Clin Infect Dis. 2011;53(10):994–1002. https://doi.org/10.1093/cid/cir632.

MIX
Papier aus verantwortungsvollen Quellen
Paper from responsible sources
FSC® C105338

If you have any concerns about our products,
you can contact us on
ProductSafety@springernature.com

In case Publisher is established outside the EU,
the EU authorized representative is:
Springer Nature Customer Service Center GmbH
Europaplatz 3, 69115 Heidelberg, Germany

Printed by Libri Plureos GmbH
in Hamburg, Germany